# ADDITIONAL TITLES FOR NEW PARENTS FROM THE AMERICAN ACADEMY OF PEDIATRICS

Baby and Toddler Basics: Expert Answers to Parents' Top 150 Questions

The CALM Baby Method: Solutions for Fussy Days and Sleepless Nights

Caring for Your Baby and Young Child: Birth to Age 5*

Dad to Dad: Parenting Like a Pro

Guide to Toilet Training

Heading Home With Your Newborn: From Birth to Reality

High Five Discipline: Positive Parenting for Happy, Healthy,
Well-Behaved Kids

My Child Is Sick! Expert Advice for Managing Common Illnesses and Injuries

The New Baby Blueprint: Caring for You and Your Little One

New Mother's Guide to Breastfeeding

Raising an Organized Child: 5 Steps to Boost Independence, Ease Frustration,
and Promote Confidence

Raising Twins: Parenting Multiples From Pregnancy
Through the School Years

Retro Baby: Timeless Activities to Boost Development–
Without All the Gear!

Sleep: What Every Parent Needs to Know

Understanding the NICU: What Parents of Preemies and Other Hospitalized
Newborns Need to Know

The Working Mom Blueprint: Winning at Parenting
Without Losing Yourse'

Your Baby's First Year

D0291155

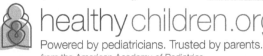

healthy children.org

Powered by pediatricians. Trusted by parents.
from the American Academy of Pediatrics

For additional parenting resources, visit the HealthyChildren bookstore at
https://shop.aap.org/for-parents.

*This book is also available in Spanish.

# Return to You

## A Postpartum Plan for New Moms

*Natasha K. Sriraman, MD, MPH, FAAP*

American Academy of Pediatrics
DEDICATED TO THE HEALTH OF ALL CHILDREN®

## American Academy of Pediatrics Publishing Staff

Mary Lou White, *Chief Product and Services Officer/SVP, Membership, Marketing, and Publishing*
Mark Grimes, *Vice President, Publishing*
Holly Kaminski, *Editor, Consumer Publishing*
Shannan Martin, *Production Manager, Consumer Publications*
Sara Hoerdeman, *Marketing Manager, Consumer Products*

Published by the American Academy of Pediatrics
345 Park Blvd
Itasca, IL 60143
Telephone: 630/626-6000
Facsimile: 847/434-8000
www.aap.org

The American Academy of Pediatrics is an organization of 67,000 primary care pediatricians, pediatric medical subspecialists, and pediatric surgical specialists dedicated to the health, safety, and well-being of all infants, children, adolescents, and young adults.

The information contained in this publication should not be used as a substitute for the medical care and advice of your pediatrician. There may be variations in treatment that your pediatrician may recommend based on individual facts and circumstances.

Statements and opinions expressed are those of the author and not necessarily those of the American Academy of Pediatrics.

Any websites, brand names, products, or manufacturers are mentioned for informational and identification purposes only and do not imply an endorsement by the American Academy of Pediatrics (AAP). The AAP is not responsible for the content of external resources. Information was current at the time of publication.

The publishers have made every effort to trace the copyright holders for borrowed materials. If they have inadvertently overlooked any, they will be pleased to make the necessary arrangements at the first opportunity.

This publication has been developed by the American Academy of Pediatrics. The contributors are expert authorities in the field of pediatrics. No commercial involvement of any kind has been solicited or accepted in the development of the content of this publication. Disclosures: The author reports no disclosures.

Every effort is made to keep *Return to You: A Postpartum Plan for New Moms* consistent with the most recent advice and information available from the American Academy of Pediatrics.

Special discounts are available for bulk purchases of this publication. Email Special Sales at nationalaccounts@aap.org for more information.

Printed in the United States of America

9-473    1 2 3 4 5 6 7 8 9 10
CB0129
ISBN: 978-1-61002-594-2
eBook: 978-1-61002-597-3
EPUB: 978-1-61002-595-9

Cover design by Daniel Rembert
Cover and publication design by Peg Mulcahy
Library of Congress Control Number: 2021913037

# What People Are Saying About
## *Return to You*

Dr Sriraman offers new parents a wonderfully comprehensive and much-needed resource for this challenging time in their lives. With sensitivity and compassion, Dr Sriraman addresses the complex variables that contribute to a new mother's vulnerability. The reader will feel empowered by the soothing, personal tone along with the evidenced-based strategies for support. *Return to You* is packed with essential information and should be handed to every single new mother and father.

> Karen Kleiman, founding director, The Postpartum Stress Center, and author of *Good Moms Have Scary Thoughts* and numerous books on postpartum depression and anxiety

Compassionate, validating, honest, and evidence-based, Dr Sriraman skillfully outlines practical guidance to moms and moms-to-be. As a pioneer of maternal mental health in the US, I am absolutely delighted to recommend *Return to You* to all my pregnant and postpartum clients.

> Shoshana S. Bennett, PhD, clinical psychologist and author of *Postpartum Depression for Dummies*

As a mother who battled postpartum depression, this book is something I wish I had read before I delivered. Dr Sriraman's approach to honest, science-based information is expertly combined with real-life experience and knowledge. This is an eye-opening read on the fourth trimester and the discrepancies we face and how to become your own advocate.

> Kristen Crowley, CPT, working mom of 2, television host, and entrepreneur

An intentionally culturally sensitive guide for parents from a source everyone can trust: a pediatrician and a mom who's seen it all personally and professionally. *Return to You* takes preparing for early parenthood to a new level.

> Whitney Casares, MD, MPH, FAAP, author of *The Working Mom Blueprint*

Moms should pack this as an essential in their hospital bag! Finally, there's a book dedicated to the profound mental, physical, and social changes new moms experience in the months following childbirth.

Having cared for thousands of moms and their children, Dr Sriraman speaks as a pediatrician and mom of 3, sharing honest perspectives, medical guidance, and sage mom advice to help navigate those intense postpartum months. From the stethoscope and the heart, she offers insights on topics you don't find in other resources—cultural approaches to postpartum, mom guilt, social media, breastfeeding, partner expectations, rights on the job, mood, anxiety disorders, and so much more.

> Sharon Cindrich, MPAL, author of the column *Plugged In Parent* and *E-Parenting: Keeping Up With Your Tech-Savvy Kids*

I love this book! Dr Sriraman's new book *Return to Me* is filled with extremely practical advice for new mothers. She gives excellent clinical guidance, peppered with personal anecdotes that make the book fun to read. She covers important postpartum topics such as fourth trimester, dealing with partner support and cultural issues, mama boundaries, handling visitors, postpartum depression, and so much more. I highly recommend this book!

> Susan Landers, MD, FAAP, FABM, author of *So Many Babies: My Life Balancing a Busy Medical Career and Motherhood*

This book is like a coffee cup conversation of exploration and truth telling between mothers, only Dr Sriraman is both a mother and a medical expert in infant care and breastfeeding, talking with you as your BFF.

> Robert M. Lawrence, MD, FABM, coeditor and coauthor of *Breastfeeding: A Guide for the Medical Profession* and adjunct clinical professor of pediatrics, University of Florida College of Medicine

As a colleague of Dr Sriraman's for more than a decade and as a reproductive psychiatrist who works exclusively with pregnant and parenting persons, it is fantastic to know that Dr Sriraman's practical and evidence-based approach to the postpartum period will now be available to all parents.

When I read this book I hear Dr Sriraman's calm, practical, and reassuring voice explaining to parenting couples what I have heard her say so many times to patients, trainees, and audiences over the past decade. I am so thankful that more parents will benefit from her advice, explanations, and perspective.

> Christine Truman, MD, reproductive psychiatrist at Partners in Women's Mental Health and assistant professor, community faculty track, Department of Psychiatry and Behavioral Sciences, Eastern Virginia Medical School

To all the mothers who have trusted me to
care for their babies over the
last 20 years.

To all the mothers who have confided in and
trusted me with their
worries, concerns, and fears.

While motherhood can be joyous, it can also
be difficult and scary.
Mamas, this book is dedicated to you.

# Equity, Diversity, and Inclusion Statement

The American Academy of Pediatrics is committed to principles of equity, diversity, and inclusion in its publishing program. Editorial boards, author selections, and author transitions (publication succession plans) are designed to include diverse voices that reflect society as a whole. Editor and author teams are encouraged to actively seek out diverse authors and reviewers at all stages of the editorial process. Publishing staff are committed to promoting equity, diversity, and inclusion in all aspects of publication writing, review, and production.

# Contents

# Acknowledgments

This book has been a labor of love since August 2019 (also known as pre-COVID times). Being a pediatrician definitely did not prepare me for motherhood, and each pregnancy, each birth, was a different experience for me. I realized that the support I needed but was unable to get truly affected me on a very deep level, as both a mother and a pediatrician. It was important for me to help not only the mothers I saw in my practice every day but to also reach mothers via speaking, researching, and blogging.

First and foremost, I would like to thank my mentor, friend, and fellow pediatrician, Karen Remley, for giving me that final push to turn my years of stories and experiences into a book. She told me that my message was very important and it needed to reach mothers and mothers-to-be everywhere.

I would also like to thank Mary Lou White, chief products and services officer/SVP, Membership, Marketing, and Publishing, for taking the time to be the first sounding board and listening to my book idea. I was so grateful for her excitement, as that helped me believe in the importance of this book. I would also like to extend my sincere gratitude for a meeting I had in fall 2019 where I met Mark Grimes, vice president, Publishing, and Barrett Winston, senior manager, Publishing acquisitions and business development, where they told me that this book was needed as it would fill a great void. I am so grateful to all 3 for being excited about the vision of my book and felt supported by their clear guidance on how to make it happen. I would also like to thank Shannan Martin, production manager, consumer publications, and Jeff Mahony, senior director, Professional and Consumer Publishing, for their shared ideas when we had our initial (virtual) meeting in spring 2020. The support and excitement from the American Academy of Pediatrics (AAP) Publishing team really helped me believe in myself.

From this meeting, I met the amazing woman who would be my editor, the fabulous Holly Kaminski. Truly, even though it was through a computer screen, her excitement was infectious. As a mother, she not only believed in the importance of this book but told me that every woman would need my book as part of her baby shower gift; the message was that important. Thank you, Holly, not only for keeping me on task, helping me to stick to deadlines, and texting me reminders; your viewpoint as a woman and a mother really helped me broaden this book through my own personal stories and the stories of all the mothers who have confided in me through all these years.

I would like to thank the AAP pediatrician reviewers from the following groups who took the time to review my manuscript:

Committee on the Fetus and Newborn

Committee on Nutrition

Committee on Psychosocial Aspects of Child and Family Health

Mental Health Leadership Work Group

Section on Breastfeeding

Task Force on Sudden Infant Death Syndrome

Your comments and suggestions continued to strengthen the message of the book. Also, thanks to Kathleen Hobson Davis, LSW, who served as a parent reviewer.

I would like to thank Sara Hoerdeman, marketing manager, consumer products, not only for her great ideas to market my book; her support of this book as a fellow mother continued to show me how important my book would be for so many mothers. I look forward to meeting the entire AAP team in person post-pandemic! I would also like to extend my thanks to my publicist Courtney Greenhalgh.

On a personal note, I would like to thank Mrs James, our very first nanny, who became another grandmother to my first 2 babies. I don't think I could have left my baby with anyone else during those early months as I drove to work sobbing. Even after she moved back to India, she continued to shower my children with love. And to Archana, her daughter, who came to our family after my son was born. She was such a core part of our family and, honestly, was my right hand as we raised (and potty trained) 2 toddlers while sleep training an infant. I can honestly say my husband and I would not have been able to do it without these 2 amazing women; "thank you" is definitely not enough.

After we moved to Virginia, not sure how we were so lucky, but Eleni came into our lives before my youngest turned 2. If you ask my kids, she is their big sister, but I consider her their second mom. We are so thankful for her as she has been an integral part of our family. Without her, I never would have been able to pursue my career in academic medicine while continuing to see patients... plus having date nights with my husband! She has been there for all 5 of us through some of the most difficult times as well as the most joyous times. Watching her now as a mother is an amazing source of happiness for me—for all of us. Eleni, thank you.

I would like to thank one of my closest friends, Sharon, for always rooting for me. She radiates so much joy and positivity. Not only did she read my initial book proposal and contract, but whatever time, day or night, I could ask her advice on book covers, color schemes, and titles. Knowing me as a mother and physician, she helped keep me focused on the message of this book and to keep that central in mind as I was writing and rewriting. And most importantly, she was always the first one to remind me to take the advice I give mamas in my practice; that is, before I can take care of my family and patients, I need to put on my oxygen mask first. Sharon, my non–MCAT-taker pal and running partner, thank you.

A special shout-out to my kids throughout this process: Sahara (who always reminds me that she is the one who made me a mother), Ishan, and Ahalya. They were always excited to hear about the book—so much so that I had to remind them not to tell their friends or post about it, as it was a work in progress. Even though they are teenagers/young adults, they will always be my babies. While I always wanted to be a mother, we all know it isn't always fun and games. Whether it's the early infant years (which are a blur), the toddler years, or adolescence, I know I made mistakes along the way (and will continue to do so). But my kids show me every day the true meaning of unconditional love. It is truly amazing to watch them grow into these responsible and caring people. To Sriraman Kids, I love you guys so very much. #ControlledChaos

And finally, last but not least, I would like to thank my husband of 24 years. He is truly my rock. Through it all, he has always believed in me. He is the first one to tell folks about a TV appearance or an article I've published and even told a friend (!!) about the book I was writing. Even when I think I can't do it, he tells me I can...no matter what. He is such an incredible father who always puts his family first.

It is truly a blessing to know that I have someone who will always have my back. I am grateful to have a partner like him on this journey of marriage and parenthood; we often laugh incredulously about how we did what we did with 2 very demanding careers. Here's to sitting on the beach one day with little umbrellas in our drinks. I love you, Raj.

Whether you are reading this book or have gifted this book to a mother who would benefit from it, *thank you*, truly, from the bottom of my heart. Whether you are a mother-to-be, a new mom, or a seasoned mom, I hope this book offers you the advice, evidence and support to help you through your postpartum journey. And it is my sincere hope that the stories I tell and the examples I use will make you feel at ease, as though you're talking to a friend. Many, many thanks, शुक्रिया.

"Be the change you wish to see in this world." -Gandhi

# Introduction

MOTHER/noun /moth·er/: a woman in relation to her child or children

When I gave birth to my first child, I was 30 years old. I was also a pediatrician, and I felt like I knew everything I needed to know going into my first delivery. Even now, I remember a nurse came and wheeled me and my now 19-year-old daughter to the front door of the hospital. It was time to go home already. At that moment, someone snapped a photo of me. In that photograph, I am sitting holding my newborn in the lobby, waiting for my husband to pull the car around. And I was crying. When people see that photograph, everyone always says, "Oh my gosh, that picture is so special." While everyone sees the poignancy of that photo, I actually remember how terrified I was at that moment. I had just given birth to my beautiful daughter and now they were pushing me out of the hospital with a brand-new human being. Even though I had just completed 3 years of pediatric residency, I was scared and overwhelmed because I honestly felt so ill-prepared for this momentous occasion.

For me, this parenting book is not just a professional endeavor; it is a personal one. This is for the new mamas out there, who are either preparing for birth or who recently gave birth. What do you see when you go online to find a book on parenting and/or motherhood? Most books focus on the baby, addressing important topics such as development, nutrition, feeding, and sleeping. Although the focus on the infant is obviously important, very few books focus on the mother. In fact, I realized that these books, while focusing on infant care, often forgot a key piece of the puzzle: Mom.

Throughout my career as a pediatrician, I have always had a strong interest in maternal health. Although I didn't completely understand the intricacies of what constituted maternal health during my education and training, throughout the years I have learned so much by caring for new mothers and babies. Every single day, I am reminded about the enduring bond between a mother and her baby.

When I began researching this book, my publishers and I were shocked that there was not one book, *not one* written about the postpartum period by a medical expert. There are books, articles, and websites out there, but figuring out what is opinion and what is fact can be challenging. And overwhelming. I am here to tell you, it's not the quantity but the quality of what you read. I promise you that everything in this book is evidence based, medically sound, and exactly what I tell my moms in practice every day.

For me, everything as a new mother was a blur. I, like many mothers, was just trying to survive and get through the day. And while there are some wonderfully amazing moments, we also have to acknowledge the difficult times, when it takes every ounce of strength to care for your infant that day, that week. My postpartum visits with the obstetrician were fast and focused on my healing and how fast my body could return to functioning as a mother and wife. My child's pediatric visits were, obviously, focused on the growth and development of the baby. I was never asked how I was feeling, how I was adjusting. No one was really focused on me, the mother. And in all fairness, during our medical training all those years ago, that is what we were taught. We focused on the immediate physical health of both mom and baby.

As a new mom, you have spent the past 9 months wondering about your baby. Who will your baby look like; will it be a boy or a girl? What color hair will the baby have, or will the baby have any at all? As a new mother, you can't wait to cuddle with your newborn and to count all the fingers and toes. You want to kiss and smell the baby and wrap him or her up tightly. My guess is that with all those thoughts and images, you probably didn't think too much about yourself, did you? Did you think about how tired you would be, or who you would ask for help in those early days if you needed it? As new moms, we begin to think of everything our child needs, while pushing our own needs aside.

In popular culture, movies, and social media, motherhood looks easy, often glorified, right? Mothers are often bombarded with advice and images on what a mother is *supposed* to look like and what she is *supposed* to be doing with her baby. Whether it is the onslaught of magazines in the grocery checkout line or the perfect images on social media, we see moms in their prepregnancy jeans, hair done, looking all put together while juggling a newborn. However, what we often don't see are the images of new mothers as they struggle.

For me, this book is a way to help normalize this aspect of motherhood, where many mothers may feel lost or inadequate, as if they're not good enough. Whether I was going from examining room to examining room visiting my patients and their new babies or speaking around the country, I saw and heard from mothers of all ages, races, religions, and backgrounds who were reaching out for help. These mothers shared their stories with me, of how they struggled, how they were embarrassed or afraid to ask for help. I am here to tell you that you are *not* alone.

# WHAT IS THE FOURTH TRIMESTER?

> **TRIMESTER**/noun /trī'mestər/: a period of 3 months, especially as a division of the duration of pregnancy

A trimester is defined as a period of 3 months, which helps mark the various stages of pregnancy. Each stage is marked with its own set of milestones as mom and baby are continually monitored during the pregnancy. Many mothers-to-be read books about pregnancy that tell them various things about the growing baby based on the weeks of pregnancy. Various apps track pregnancy and capture special moments. As the mom and baby grow, customary celebrations mark different stages of the pregnancy. Whether it is a surprise baby shower, a gender reveal, a maternity photo shoot, or a "baby-moon" with your significant other (or even all of them!), pregnancy is generally an exciting time for mamas to be. As it should be!

However, once the baby is delivered, there are 2 of you. For the past 3 trimesters, a mother has become one with this baby, forming an intense physical and psychological connection. Thinking of 2 people but taking care of one body. Just because the baby is now outside the womb does not mean that mom and baby are no longer connected. In fact, in some ways you are now even more connected to your infant.

Why is the fourth trimester so important to me? Because as a mother and pediatrician, I am in the position to offer evidence-based information along with real-life advice. It doesn't matter how many books you read or how many children you have or even if your career (like mine) revolves around babies, let me tell you this: There is no instruction manual for being a mom. Struggling with breastfeeding, feeling isolated and overwhelmed, having excessive guilt about returning to work; I had *all* of that.

I feel fortunate that my professional passion and my personal experiences allow me to help new moms and their families as they navigate the postpartum period. While having a baby is supposed to be the happiest time of your life, for some it isn't. And for many, it is the most challenging.

## My Mantra

I want all my mamas to know this: I want all my mamas to know this:

- It is OK to ask for help.
- It is OK not to do it all.
- It is OK to want to take a break.
- It is OK to talk to your doctor if you're not feeling well.

Remember, once the baby is born, so is a new mother. We often forget to care for and nurture mama. We often forget to ask mom how *she* is doing. My mantra that I always tell mamas is this: *Happy and healthy mama equals happy and healthy baby.*

Whether you received this book from your best friend or from a family member, just know this: I wrote this book for *you* mama. A woman who is incredible, strong, and resilient, a woman who has not only carried but nurtured a human being. As you care for your baby, I want you to know that you too deserve to be taken care of and nurtured. Whether the issue is physical, emotional, personal, or professional, I will address each of these, and more, in the ensuing chapters. As you continue to care for your newborn, I hope you find that this book empowers you on your journey of motherhood. Thank you for trusting me on that journey.

# History of Postpartum Care

When I was a pediatric resident, I knew that I wanted to wait to have a family, even though I was married, because my grueling call schedule made it too difficult to manage a new baby while taking care of my professional responsibilities. During my month in the neonatal intensive care unit, I remember working with a younger resident, also married, who was from a European country. She told me, "I'm not having a baby until I'm done with residency and I can move back home. I will have a lot more help and time off after delivering over there." Back then, even though I didn't know the significance of what she told me, I still remember it clearly.

## POSTPARTUM PERIOD

First of all, let's define the *postpartum period.* While it means after childbirth, whether we discuss it within a medical context (your postpartum visit with the obstetrician) or a personal context (postpartum leave), many people, including me, define the immediate postpartum period as that 3-month period after the birth of your baby—in other words, your fourth trimester.

What did my colleague mean when she said that? After I had my baby, why was it that my relatives from India were shocked at what my postpartum period looked like?

Why do so many of my patients from other countries tell me it's harder to have a baby in this country?

When thinking about this book, I felt it was important to talk about what postpartum looks like, not just in the United States, but also in different parts of the world. The United States spends more money per person on health care than other developed countries, but our health outcomes for mothers and babies rank much lower than those of other wealthy nations. Why is that? One major reason is that postpartum care in the United States is, frankly, disgraceful.

Birth may signal the end of a woman's pregnancy, but it is only the beginning of so much more. The postpartum period is often not recognized as being vital to the health and well-being of both mom and baby.

When I spoke at a conference in the Philippines in 2019 about breastfeeding and postpartum depression, the audience, composed of physicians, nurses, and other health care providers who worked with mama-baby dyads, was shocked to hear that new mothers in the United States have their first obstetrician postpartum visit 6 weeks after delivery. Honestly, there was a collective gasp in that room of around 1,000 people.

On a professional level, I see a vast difference for my mothers who have had children in their native countries as well as in the United States. For instance, the level of support from family members and the community is different from the pressures placed on mothers in the United States. Every day I see mothers who, for financial and familial reasons, are going back to work or school within 6 weeks after delivery; I've actually seen mothers going back to work within 2 weeks. On a personal level, I witnessed the differences for my family and friends who had babies in India versus the United States and their expectations as to the amount of help they would receive on arriving home with their newborn. In many countries and societies around the world, it truly is a village that helps mom when she returns home with her newborn.

## TRADITIONS IN OTHER COUNTRIES

What do other countries do to help their mothers during the fourth trimester?

One of the most common traditions in countries around the world is something called the *40-day lying in period.* This has also been referred to as *postpartum confinement.* Before thinking this is crazy or not for you, let me explain how this helps moms and their babies during this particularly stressful time.

In India, the 40- to 60-day period, known as *jaappa* in Hindi, allows mom to stay home and rest while preventing her and the baby from being exposed to any type of infection. In Pakistan, this postpartum tradition is known as *sawa mahina*, meaning 5 weeks. The only thing for mom to do is rest and nourish (breastfeed) the baby. Mom is fed nourishing foods, cooked by family members, that are easily digestible and meant to keep her body warm. After having my second child, our nanny, who had emigrated from India many years earlier, was with me during those early weeks helping care for my oldest child (a toddler in diapers). She just could not understand why I was still doing things around the house; my husband was back to work within a week and we had no help from our families. Regardless of what she was doing to keep my toddler occupied, she tried to get me to eat well instead of snacking when I had time. I still remember the protein-rich dish she gave me made with herbs that not only nourished me but actually helped increase my breast milk. Ironically, as I learned later on while studying to become an IBCLC (International Board Certified Lactation Consultant) and starting my own breastfeeding medicine practice, I realized that the herb she used, *methi*—known in Western countries as fenugreek—is a common galactogogue that mothers can take to help increase breast milk production.

In China, the postpartum recovery period is sometimes referred to as sitting the month; during this time, new mothers are advised to stay inside to recover and focus on feeding their newborn. Aspects of Chinese medicine are included to nourish mom while increasing her breast milk supply. In some areas, visitors are not allowed for the first 12 days. Mothers are also discouraged from bathing, washing their hair, or having any contact with cold weather as this may increase their risk of catching a cold. In some, more modern areas, after mothers shower, they must dry off immediately and can use a hair dryer to help keep warm. Similar to other cultures, preparation of food in China is an important aspect of postpartum healing. Mothers are given easily digestible foods rich in protein that are prepared by female family members. These foods give mom energy while helping to shrink the uterus and facilitating physical healing.

In Korea, postpartum confinement is known as *sanhujori*, which can last from 1 week to 1 month. Mothers eat healthy food and perform easy exercises that help warm the body, which allows for physical recovery. While these services were previously provided by family members, they are now provided by various postpartum centers and workers who can come into the home. Services include anything from skin therapy and body massage to full-time help caring for the newborn. The goal is to help mom heal completely, both physically and mentally, not only to help her prepare for any future pregnancies, but also to prevent health conditions that can negatively affect her later in life, such as joint issues, incontinence, and depression. Clearly, the need is there, as more than 50% of mothers in Korea use these services.

Among many Latina mothers, *la cuarentena* helps them ease into the transition of motherhood. *Cuarentena* lasts about 40 days or 6 weeks (do you see the pattern?) during which she focuses on her physical healing and caring for and nourishing her newborn by breastfeeding. Members of the extended family take care of cooking, cleaning, and caring for any older children. Depending on the family, the type and consistency of foods are a central part of the mother's postpartum healing process.

So while we focus on birth plans, baby showers, and gender reveals in the United States, other countries start discussing and teaching about postpartum care to help women while they are still pregnant. For example, in the Netherlands, mothers begin planning for their postpartum period at 33 weeks' gestation. In Spain, pregnant women receive their own mother's passport called the *cartilla de embarazo*. They take this passport with them as they are tended to by a community midwife each month, not just for prenatal baby care, but also to start planning for the immediate postpartum period.

In Germany, a woman receives a booklet called a *mutterpass* at her first prenatal appointment. Not only does it track her prenatal visits, but mom continues to present it at all her postpartum visits so that all health issues, for both mom and baby, can be tracked and followed during pregnancy and the postpartum period. This eases the transition into the fourth trimester, allowing care for mom to continue and remain consistent.

Probably the best known maternity package around the world comes from Finland. Remember when Kate, Duchess of Cambridge, received a gift from the Finnish Government? What was in this special package? Once mothers are 154 days into their pregnancy (approximately 22 weeks' gestation), they can apply for a free baby box through the country's social security system. This box is available to all mothers, regardless of financial or employment status. Although the colorful box is filled with essentials for the baby, such as diapers, baby toiletries, clothing, and a book, it also contains a small mattress, so it can double as an initial bed for the baby, almost like a bassinette. Not only is this helpful to many moms, but this baby box emphasizes the importance of placing the newborn on a flat surface to sleep. This practice has also been shown to be effective in lowering infant mortality rates in Finland.

As these examples illustrate, postpartum care around the world varies greatly, but one common theme exists. Mothers are taken care of not only during their pregnancy, but also after delivery as they enter the postpartum period. While babies are being cared for by their mothers, family members and others in the community are focused on caring for mom's physical and mental well-being.

To all the mothers who are reading this book, postpartum practices from different areas of the world do impact us directly in the United States. Whether you emigrated from another country or have family members in other parts of the world who come here to help once the baby is born, we will see an overlap of these various postpartum practices that will impact what the fourth trimester looks like for you and your baby.

And to my mothers from the United States or other Western societies who may not have postpartum cultural or familial practices, perhaps the information in this book will help you start to construct the ideal postpartum journey based on what you need.

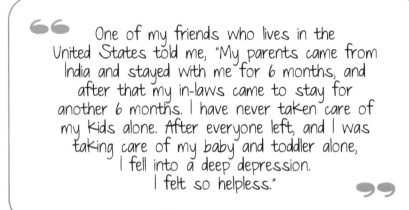

" One of my friends who lives in the United States told me, "My parents came from India and stayed with me for 6 months, and after that my in-laws came to stay for another 6 months. I have never taken care of my kids alone. After everyone left, and I was taking care of my baby and toddler alone, I fell into a deep depression. I felt so helpless." "

In the next chapter, I will explore postpartum care in the United States and how it affects mom and baby. My hope is that you, whether pregnant or a new mom, will gain the information you need to move into your fourth trimester feeling empowered and confident.

# CHAPTER 2

# Current State of Postpartum Care

> **POSTPARTUM**/adjective/pōs(t)-ˈpär-təm: occurring in or being the period following childbirth

*N*ow that we have taken a glimpse into what postpartum care looks like in other parts of the world, let's take a closer look at postpartum practices here in the United States.

As a pediatrician for the past 20 plus years and a mom for the past 19 plus years, it has become clear to me that postpartum care in this country does not take care of the mother. The postpartum period focuses on the health and safety of the newborn, but it lacks support for the woman who just gave birth.

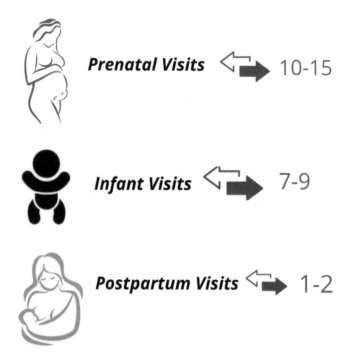

*Prenatal Visits* ⟵➡ 10-15

*Infant Visits* ⟵➡ 7-9

*Postpartum Visits* ⟵➡ 1-2

## Let's Do Some Math ... Promise, No Calculus

During a normal pregnancy (with no complications or need for extra visits), a woman is seen at least 10 to 15 times by her obstetrician.

Within the first year after delivery, pediatricians see the baby between 7 and 9 times, and this does not include any sick visits.

What about after the baby is born? When is mom seen again after this miraculous task of childbirth?

If mom has a cesarean delivery, she will be seen in 2 weeks for an incision check. At this visit, mom usually will be given clearance for small tasks or activities. For me, being able to drive was a big one.

Mothers who have had a regular vaginal delivery may not be seen until 6 weeks afterward.

Yes, you heard that correctly. Six weeks! I always find it crazy that after such close follow-up of a mom's physical and mental health during the pregnancy that after giving birth, she is left to figure it out and fend for herself until the 6-week visit.

It has always been interesting to me that when a mom brings her baby to me for those frequent newborn visits and weight checks, they often ask what they should do about their episiotomy pain, leg swelling, or overwhelming anxiety ... just to name a few concerns.

The American College of Obstetricians and Gynecologists (ACOG) addressed this issue by stressing the importance of tailoring the postpartum plan to each mom. Moms need to be seen sooner than 6 weeks' postpartum and more frequently. One size does not fit all. The ACOG statement, "Optimizing Postpartum Care," was developed as a result of concerns about complications faced by many mothers after childbirth. For more information, visit https://www.acog.org/clinical/clinical-guidance/committee-opinion/articles/2018/05/optimizing-postpartum-care.

More than 700 women die every year in the United States from causes related to pregnancy and childbirth, with more than 50,000 women experiencing life-threatening complications after delivery. These statistics are among the worst compared to those in other industrialized countries. Sadly, Black mothers are 3 to 4 times more likely to die than White mothers. In addition to bias in health care, the lack of timely responses to patient concerns and lack of safety measures contribute to this statistic. The evidence shows that continuous support during labor and the postpartum period results in improved outcomes for both mom and baby.

## WHAT HAPPENS AFTER DELIVERY?

Regardless of the type of delivery a woman has had, she is generally discharged within 3 to 4 days. I wrote this book during the COVID-19 pandemic, and moms were being discharged home with their babies as early as 26 hours after giving birth! Unfortunately, issues that mom may be having are not always addressed while she is in the hospital. Also, issues often don't even arise until mom is home. Unless the issue is emergent or mom calls her obstetrician, it won't be addressed until she sees her doctor in 6 weeks. As I write this down, it sounds ridiculous, no?

I remember leaving the hospital on the fourth day after my first cesarean delivery. After checking that my daughter's car seat met the requirements, the nurse discharging me told me not to have sex for the next 6 weeks, and my obstetrician would clear me at my 6-week postpartum visit. That was it. I honestly just stared at her blankly and chuckled at the incredulity of that statement. For various reasons, moms and their newborns are discharged quickly in the United States, and because of these speedy discharges, moms often do not receive the help or advice they need. As a new mom, you are sent home with a packet of information, which, let's be honest, isn't that helpful when you're going home with a brand new human being. Short hospital stays and inadequate maternity support do a disservice to our mothers.

> 66 A mother who brought her newborn to my office for the first visit wanted to breastfeed but was having difficulty. She told me, "I didn't even see a lactation consultant while I was in the hospital since I was discharged by the weekend. My milk started coming in after I got home and I tried calling the hospital warm line, but it wasn't helpful." 99

After months of frequent visits with an obstetrician, a single 6-week postpartum checkup does a disservice to all our mothers, many of whom may be experiencing various issues, ranging from breastfeeding problems to physical pain after delivery and mental health issues. This large gap of time during which mothers are not seen by their obstetricians can lead to complications if issues and concerns are not addressed in a timely fashion. In addition to the physical complications, this delay often leaves moms feeling hopeless and helpless as they try to find help on their own.

Because moms see their pediatrician quickly and more frequently than their obstetrician, I am often fielding mom's questions during the newborn visits, which is fine. I feel fortunate that these women feel comfortable enough to tell me about their physical discomfort or the sadness they've been feeling. Although I want all mamas to reach out and ask for help, it is essential to reach out to a physician or other professional who is accessible without delay. That includes your baby's pediatrician. But this is not a solution.

## WHY DOES THIS HAPPEN?

While obstetricians, pediatricians, doulas, and midwives who work with mothers and babies realize that this model is neither safe nor healthy, this gap in postpartum care is not dictated or decided by physicians or other health care professionals. Follow-up care is dictated by insurance companies, which (at least in the United States) decide the timing and frequency of postpartum obstetrical visits. Although medical organizations can make recommendations, the final decision is not ours to make. While there are postpartum doulas and home-visiting services, they may not be readily available, easy to navigate, or affordable. One of the most powerful statements I heard after the release of ACOG's statement about ideal postpartum care is this: *The baby is the candy, the mom is the wrapper, and once the candy is out of the wrapper, the wrapper is cast aside.* Sadly, in countries with poor postpartum resources and support, this is often how many mothers feel ... completely tossed aside and forgotten about.

Despite the barriers, there is still hope. Because of my personal and professional experiences, I realized that postpartum care for the mother needs to be repackaged and redefined. So although we define pregnancy in terms of trimesters, the mom–baby connection does not end once the baby is born. The baby is still connected to you, mother, and just like in the womb, the newborn still needs you for protection, well–being, and nourishment. This postpartum period is often referred to as the fourth trimester, which is the 12-week period immediately after you have had the baby. Even though not all mothers have heard of this term, every mother and newborn will go through it.

In addition, just because the support is not defined or adequately covered by health insurance, this does not mean that you can't prepare for your fourth trimester. As you move through this book, you'll find examples that can help you prepare for your baby's delivery. Chapter 4 describes how to create your own postpartum plan to assist you as you prepare for the physical and mental changes that naturally occur after delivery. The goal is to start planning while you're pregnant.

With this book, I want to change how mothers experience their postpartum journey. I want your journey to be positive. I want you to feel empowered during this journey.

As we plan for the baby with showers, gender reveals, and baby registries, we need to keep in mind that motherhood is so much more than pregnancy and the birth. I am a firm believer that gathering information and planning ahead will help moms navigate, prepare, and enjoy the fourth trimester—all of it. It isn't always easy, but I hope I can make the transition into the postpartum period a bit easier for mothers.

CHAPTER 3

# You're Pregnant... Now What?

PREGNANT /adjective/'pregnənt/): (of a woman or female animal) having a child or young developing in the uterus

> " I bought a pregnancy test and went into the bathroom. I don't know who was more nervous, me or my husband. Did we really only wait a few minutes? It seemed much longer. When I saw the 2 lines, I showed my husband the evidence that he was going to be a father. Even 20 years later, I will never forget his reaction. Tears, excitement, nervousness. After I sat him down on the couch when he became a little light-headed, he said, "I need to start a college account!" "

## YOU'RE PREGNANT

Congratulations! You're pregnant! Whether it's a visit to the doctor or peeing on a stick, you have confirmation you are pregnant and are ecstatic. So, what's next? There are probably a million thoughts running through your head right now... not to mention your partner's. It seems like a whirlwind. You are feeling overwhelmed, excited, and nervous. Although you don't need to start planning for college immediately after peeing on the stick, you probably are starting to make a planning list in your head once you've come off cloud 9. It is 100% under-standable to start planning and thinking ahead as you move through your pregnancy. However, as you have read, although many aspects of the pregnancy are necessary (as well as fun), they don't always prepare you for the baby you will be returning home with.

I was prompted to write this book in large part because of my own experiences as a new mom, as well as what I continue to see as a pediatrician in my daily interactions with newborns and their moms.

### New Moms' Reactions After Delivery

As a pediatrician, I see new moms and their babies in my office for the first checkup at 1 week old. It is the first time I get to ask the new moms how they are doing and feeling, while also examin-ing the newborns. Typical comments are:

- No one ever told me how hard this would be.
- I wasn't expecting it to be like this.
- I thought breastfeeding would be easy.
- I have never felt this tired in my entire life.
- Everyone makes it look so easy. I must be doing it wrong.

I remember going through my first pregnancy, the excitement about starting this next chapter of our lives. Thrilled to see my baby on a black-and-white screen (no 4-dimensional sonograms back then). Sharing the sonogram photos with friends and family. Worried and shocked when I was put on bed rest. Frustrated when I received such little support from my employer. Overwhelmed as I was showered with gifts at the baby shower, wondering if I was really supposed to use all of this stuff.

The hospital then sent me home with a newborn, a human being, after only 4 days. Really? It didn't matter that I had been babysitting since I was 11 years old. It didn't matter that I became a big sister at the age of 14. And it definitely didn't matter that I was a newly minted pediatrician. Nothing I read prepared me for those early days of being a mother.

Honestly, I liken it to wedding festivities: the bridal shower, bachelorette party, and wedding. Fun, right? Of course! But did all those parties and the ceremony prepare you for marriage? Of course not! Marriage is fun, but there are ups and downs, challenges and celebrations.

Hence, my primary reason for writing this book is that pregnancy and all the preparations for baby do not adequately prepare us for motherhood. A friend commented, "I read every book out there when I was pregnant. I knew everything about being pregnant. Then the hospital sent me home with my baby and I had absolutely no idea what to do!" She was 100% correct.

I want this book to provide you with a road map so you will be prepared for those days after you arrive home with your newborn.

As you prepare the nursery and register for the shower, let me help you develop a strategy to prepare for motherhood *while* pregnant. As a pediatrician, I will always focus on evidence-based information. As a mother, I will offer advice that is realistic for you and your family.

## PREPARE FOR BIRTH

First, talk to friends who have recently become mothers. This can be helpful as they have recently been pregnant and are currently *in* that postpartum period. They may be able to help guide you as you start preparations because they will know what did and did not work for them.

Second, make a list. Seriously, I love making lists and then checking things off. What will you need in those early days? What items will be important for to have both in the hospital and when you return home? You will want a list for the baby, but you also need one for yourself. These items on your list are great to put on your registry if you decide to do one.

### Prenatal Classes

Where can you attend prenatal classes that will help you prepare for childbirth? What about any breastfeeding classes in your area? Start by asking your obstetrician's office as it may have this information. Try searching locally or asking a friend or neighbor who may be familiar with local resources.

### Tour the Hospital

Will you have an opportunity to tour the hospital or birthing center? I think this is important, not only for you but also for your partner or family member who will attend the birth with you. Gaining that familiarity helps to decrease the feelings of stress and anxiety due to not knowing what to expect. Also, start thinking about the driving route to the hospital once contractions begin.

### Birth Doula/Postpartum Doula

Depending on the family, some mothers may hire a birth doula and/or a postpartum doula to provide additional help during the delivery and immediate postpartum period. A doula is a woman, without formal obstetrical training, who is employed to provide guidance and support to a pregnant woman during labor and can also provide postpartum support once mother and baby go home.

Many doulas serve in both roles, whereas others may only cover the delivery or the postpartum period. A birth doula will be your coach during the delivery, your own personal cheerleader while helping to make the birthing process easier on you. This is not to replace your spouse, partner, or another family member who will be with you in the delivery room. Please note that during the current COVID-19 pandemic, hospitals are limiting the number of people who can be present during the delivery. So until this changes, please speak to your obstetrician or hospital regarding its policy prior to your delivery date.

A postpartum doula (or a night nurse) will come to your home after you return with your newborn and act as your right hand. Whether it's taking care of your immediate needs or feeding the baby at night so you can get some sleep, that extra level of support can be life-changing with respect to how your postpartum journey progresses. Again, while this option may be accessible to some families, this does not replace those family and friends who volunteered to be there as your support system after you return home with your newborn.

### Finding a Pediatrician

Looking for a pediatrician is important further along in your pregnancy. Often, the pediatrician who examines your baby in the hospital will not be available once you are discharged. Each area and region of the country is different. It is important to find a pediatrician who is accessible in terms of distance and office hours. You also should find out how the pediatrician's office handles after-hours calls.

### Advice and the Internet

Another aspect of managing immense amounts of information is receiving advice from others, whether this is your mother, mother-in-law, sister, aunt, or best friend. Remember: Every mama is different. Every baby is different. Every pregnancy is different. What may have worked for your work colleague or sister, and even what may have worked for you during a prior pregnancy/birth, might not work for you for this pregnancy, birth, and postpartum period.

Remember, one size does not fit all, and there is no one *right way* (whatever that means) to go through pregnancy and into your postpartum period. So, view others' advice as you would anything you read. Listen to it and file it away. Opinion does not equal fact.

While technology has given us information at our fingertips, unfortunately, the information on the internet is often incorrect. In fact, scientific studies show that women who search the internet for information related to pregnancy and infant concerns often experience anxiety and stress. You can usually find something on the internet that will support something you have heard or a symptom that you or your baby are experiencing. However, what I tell my mothers is this: Many of the Google searches or websites you go to are not offering sound medical advice. With the internet, people can post and write about almost anything, and this includes motherhood. But just because one went through a pregnancy and shared delivery and postpartum complications does not make it correct advice. The information you read can be overwhelming and frankly exhausting. Keep in mind that just because someone writes about their own experience or expresses an opinion does not make it factually correct. Much of the information and advice is not evidence based. Sadly, I see moms questioning things and worrying about their babies based on something they heard or read on the internet. Remember, as a physician, I went to school a lot longer than Dr Google. If you have any questions or concerns, bring them to the attention of your doctor. That is what they are there for.

### Fourth Trimester

Until recently, the fourth trimester had not been considered an important part of the pregnancy. Although the focus still tends to be on the 3 trimesters of pregnancy, things are changing. The medical establishment as well as society in general are becoming more aware of the importance of the postpartum period, especially its focus on the new mom. This may be different from what your family and friends experienced. However, even though others in your inner circle may not have had the opportunity to plan for the immediate postpartum period, this does not mean that you shouldn't. Planning for your postpartum period does not detract from your health and well-being during the pregnancy. In fact, postpartum planning will help you feel calmer during your pregnancy, thereby reducing stress.

I am going to guide you through construction of your very own postpartum plan (see Chapter 4). This will help both my mothers-to-be and my current mamas plan for their fourth trimester and anticipate anything that they and their babies may need. Just as any new mom packs a diaper bag with all those just in case items, having a postpartum plan in place will alleviate your worries and fears, so you too will be fully prepared.

Some of you may be reading this and wondering whether it is more important to have a birth plan in place first. A birth plan outlines your preferences during your labor and delivery. It may include things such as who will be at the delivery, whether you want pain medication, even music and lighting choices. However, the birth plan doesn't always go as planned depending on the circumstances in that moment of delivery. Anything can happen during the birthing process, and your birth plan may change based on what your physician/obstetric provider believes is safest for you and your baby. Thus, it is important to remain flexible as things can change, and sometimes quickly. So while the birth plan may be important to many pregnant women, it is one small piece of this amazing journey you are on.

So mama, enjoy your pregnancy and everything that goes with it. And as you plan and prepare, allow your family and friends to shower you with all the rituals surrounding pregnancy.

# CHAPTER 4

# Your Postpartum Plan

**PLAN**/noun/plan/: a detailed proposal for doing or achieving something

In this chapter, I will help you construct a plan to enable you to identify your support system and resources for your fourth trimester. Because no one can predict the steps in your mother-hood journey, my goal is to help you, your spouse/partner, and family prepare and plan for your needs in the immediate post-partum period.

## WHY IS A POSTPARTUM PLAN IMPORTANT?

As discussed in previous chapters, during pregnancy you are planning for the birth of your baby while enjoying the changes occurring inside you. However, as we have seen, learning and reading about pregnancy may not fully prepare you for the changes you'll encounter in the postpartum period. My goal in this chapter is for you to complete a realistic postpartum plan that will address all areas for which you need to be prepared once you deliver your baby and enter your fourth trimester. While developing this plan before your delivery will be helpful, please know that you can modify it during the postpartum period.

Let this chapter be a starting point for discussions about how you and your family will adjust to life with a new baby. I want you to have as many resources as possible at your fingertips, including a complete list that specifies where you can ask for and find help if and when you need it.

So grab your water bottle, find a comfortable place to sit, and let's get started!

### Rest

During those first few weeks and months following the birth of a baby, it is essential for mothers to get rest. I know it may sound difficult, but the aim is for mothers to get 4 to 5 hours of uninterrupted sleep at a time. Mothers will need support, whether it's during the day to nap or through the night, but sleep and rest are needed to maintain normal functioning. Use this list to start thinking about whom you can ask for help during various time periods. I want you to feel comfortable and find people you can truly rely on, such as family, friends, doulas, babysitters, community members, and/or religious groups.

Strategies on how to fill in these gaps will be discussed throughout this book.

### Support

It is important to have friends who are parents of young babies. Someone to talk to who can empathize with you, which is especially beneficial on days when you are feeling particularly overwhelmed. Friends in a similar stage of life are an important addition to your support network, your village.

If you don't have friends or neighbors with young babies, then strategize on where you can connect with these mothers if possible, such as childbirth education classes, prenatal/postnatal fitness classes, breastfeeding support groups, online discussion groups, community groups, and religious groups.

## Your Postpartum Plan

| | Name/Contact Information |
|---|---|
| People available during the day: | 1. |
| | 2. |
| | 3. |
| People available at night: | 1. |
| | 2. |
| | 3. |
| People available during evening hours (also can help with older siblings): | 1. |
| | 2. |
| | 3. |
| People available to move in to provide extra support: | 1. |
| | 2. |
| | 3. |

|  | Name/Contact Information |
| --- | --- |
| Names of friends/ neighbors with babies of their own: | 1. |
|  | 2. |
|  | 3. |
| New friends who have young children: | 1. |
|  | 2. |
|  | 3. |

## *Nutrition*

Healthy meals and adequate hydration are important for moms during the immediate postpartum period. However, eating and staying hydrated can be challenging for new moms as they care for their newborns. Holding, feeding, burping, and changing infants leaves moms with little time to eat, let alone cook. Planning meals for the fourth trimester before your baby arrives will assist you and those helping you care for the baby.

You can plan meals in advance by preparing double batches and freezing meals. Consider identifying grocery stores that can deliver to your house, as well as meal delivery services available in your neighborhood.

Ask friends, family, neighbors, and/or coworkers to help prepare, deliver, or send you family meals through various online delivery services if possible. If your friends and family members ask, let them know what kind of meals are preferred, taking into consideration any dietary restrictions and allergies. Doing so may take the burden of cooking off you and your partner.

| | Name/Contact Information |
|---|---|
| Nutritious meals to prepare and freeze before the baby arrives: | 1.<br>2.<br>3. |
| Grocery stores that offer online shopping and/or delivery: | 1.<br>2.<br>3. |
| Nutritious and affordable take-out options (eg, Uber Eats, DoorDash, Grubhub): | 1.<br>2.<br>3. |
| People who have volunteered to prepare and deliver nutritious meals after baby arrives: | 1.<br>2.<br>3. |

MealTrain.com is a web-based tool that friends and family can use to sign up for meal delivery.

## FEEDING YOUR BABY

Feeding a new baby can be a full-time job. The initial days can be especially challenging as parents and their baby figure out what works best for them. Feeding choices—breast, bottle, or both—do not need to be permanent. Some mothers prefer one technique, while others choose a hybrid approach. Whatever you decide, keep in mind that the choice is not permanent and often changes during this postpartum period. Please remember to always consult your baby's physician or health care provider regarding any questions or concerns you have about feeding your newborn and any struggles you may be experiencing.

Each and every baby is unique. Each and every situation is unique. Choose what works best for you, your baby, and your family.

### Breastfeeding

Breastfeeding is a natural process, but it does not always come naturally. I tell all breastfeeding mothers in my practice: Just because it's natural does not mean it's easy. Depending on your family and friends, many mothers lack the support they need when struggling with breastfeeding. Many women deal with painful nipples, inadequate milk supply, and concerns about their baby's weight gain, which can cause stress, worry, and guilt leading to many mothers' not meeting their breastfeeding goals. It is important to think about your breastfeeding goals while pregnant and use this plan to help line up and enlist those supports that will help you meet your goals during the fourth trimester.

Appropriate support can prevent many of these difficulties. During those first few weeks, it is important to continue breast-feeding to maintain supply. I want you to identify and line up support before those issues begin. I do not want any of my mothers to feel as if they are alone in their struggles.

## *Formula Feeding*

If formula feeding is part of your feeding goals, it is important to realize that it also consists of many aspects, including how to mix formula, what water to use, bottle options, choice of formula, how much to feed, and how often to feed.

| | Name/Contact Information |
|---|---|
| Friends and family members who will support and encourage my infant-feeding choices: | 1.<br><br>2.<br><br>3. |
| People who are informed and up-to-date about infant-feeding choices who can answer questions and make helpful recommendations: | 1.<br><br>2.<br><br>3. |
| Local postpartum doulas who will visit and help with infant feeding: | 1.<br><br>2.<br><br>3. |

| | Name/Contact Information |
|---|---|
| Local board-certified lactation consultants who will help with breastfeeding: | 1. |
| | 2. |
| | 3. |
| Local resources that provide emotional support and high-quality breastfeeding information: | 1. |
| | 2. |
| | 3. |
| Breastfeeding support groups in your community: | 1. |
| | 2. |
| | 3. |
| Evidence-based online breastfeeding support groups: | 1. |
| | 2. |
| | 3. |

| | Name/Contact Information |
|---|---|
| Places to purchase or rent breastfeeding pumps and supplies: | 1. |
| | 2. |
| | 3. |

| Resources for Feeding Your Baby | |
|---|---|
| La Leche League International | www.llli.org |
| International Lactation Consultant Association | www.ILCA.org |
| Women, Infants, and Children (WIC) | https://wicbreastfeeding.fns.usda.gov/ |
| DONA International (doula) | www.dona.org |
| Best for Babes | bestforbabes.com |

## OLDER SIBLINGS

Moms need to understand that older children will experience a time of transition following the birth of a new baby. This is a normal part of child development. Although moms want to welcome the baby with love while maintaining a loving, nurturing relationship with older children, this is not always easy. An important step to ensuring a smooth transition is to plan ahead so that older children have time to welcome their new sibling but still have special time with mom and/or dad.

| | Name/Contact Information |
|---|---|
| People who can care for my older children when I go into labor: | 1. |
| | 2. |
| | 3. |
| People who are available to spend quality time with older children (including driving them to school, child care, activities): | 1. |
| | 2. |
| | 3. |
| Special activities to share with older children (eg, playground, bike rides): | 1. |
| | 2. |
| | 3. |

## RENEWING AND RECHARGING

The time spent together as a growing family is important, but parents also need time to connect and nurture their relationship. However, accomplishing this does not happen easily or spontaneously and does require planning. Remember, it is important to find that occasional "me" and "us" time, allowing you to recharge and strengthen bonding with each other, the baby, and the family.

| | Name/Contact Information |
|---|---|
| Friends/family who can provide occasional child care: | 1. <br> 2. <br> 3. |
| Professional child care providers: | 1. <br> 2. <br> 3. |
| Activities that allow mom to rest, renew, and reenergize (eg, read, meet with friends, take exercise class): | 1. <br> 2. <br> 3. |
| Activities for social interactions (ie, connect with spouse/partner, friends, family) | 1. <br> 2. <br> 3. |

## MOM'S MENTAL HEALTH

Postpartum depression and anxiety affect up to 20% to 25% of women during pregnancy or the first year after giving birth. Mental health is one of the highest priorities during this time. Fortunately, these conditions can be treated in various ways, such as self-care, peer support, counseling, therapy, and, if necessary, medications.

Please reach out to your obstetrician or the health professional who delivered your baby if you have any questions or concerns about how you are feeling. You can also speak to your baby's health care provider, who can direct you to various resources.

| Resources for Mom's (Dad's/Partner's) Mental Health | |
|---|---|
| Postpartum Support International | www.postpartum.net |
| Substance Abuse and Mental Health Services Administration | www.samhsa.gov/find-help/national-helpline |
| Office on Women's Health | www.womenshealth.gov/mental-health/mental-health-conditions/postpartum-depression |
| MGH Center for Women's Mental Health | https://womensmentalhealth.org/ |

## Feelings of Self-harm

If you are having any thoughts of self-harm or suicide, *please* call one of the following for immediate assistance:

- 911
- National Suicide Prevention Lifeline: 1-800-273-8255
- Suicide Prevention Hotline: 1-800-SUICIDE
- National Postpartum Depression Warmline: 1-800-PPD-MOMS

| | Name/Contact Information |
|---|---|
| People who will comfort you or provide a shoulder to cry on: | 1. <br> 2. <br> 3. |
| Friends or family members to call late at night: | 1. <br> 2. <br> 3. |

|  | Name/Contact Information |
|---|---|
| Local support groups: www.postpartum.net/ get-help/locations/ | 1. |
| | 2. |
| | 3. |
| Knowledgeable mental health professionals: | 1. |
| | 2. |
| | 3. |
| Obstetrician/physician/ midwife who delivered my baby: (Office number/on-call number) | 1. |
| Baby's pediatrician/ health care provider (Office number/on-call number) | 1. |

## RETURNING TO "NORMAL"

When is your partner or spouse returning to work? Are you returning to work or school? Regardless of your family situation, identifying resources to help with the baby, older children, and household duties is important so that you are not overwhelmed by all the changes and responsibilities a new baby brings. Keep in mind, every situation is different and every family is unique. Identify what works best for you, your baby, and your family.

| | Name/Contact Information |
|---|---|
| What child care options are available? | 1. |
| | 2. |
| | 3. |
| Plan for housekeeping and chores? | 1. |
| | 2. |
| | 3. |
| What are mom's concerns about this transition? | 1. |
| | 2. |
| | 3. |
| What are the partner's concerns about this transition? | 1. |
| | 2. |
| | 3. |

"Mommy-ing" is hard. There is no one right way to do things. Do what comes naturally to you. Do what works for you, your spouse or partner, your family, and your baby. Don't hesitate to reach out to your baby's pediatrician/health care provider with any questions you have along the way.

I hope this postpartum plan helps guide you as you prepare contingency plans before the baby's arrival. I believe that planning and preparation will not only assist you in your fourth trimester, but it will also help prevent problems and challenges from escalating because you will have the resources at hand and ready to go.

Finally, always remember that it is OK to ask for help. Promise.

CHAPTER 5

# Role of the Father/Partner

> PARTNER/noun/ 'pärt-nər: a person with whom one shares an intimate relationship: one member of a couple
>
> FATHER/noun/ 'fä-thər: a male parent

Understanding the role of the father/partner/significant other after childbirth is really important. There are so many things to consider. How can your partner support you? Does your partner have his or her own relationship with the baby? What can mothers do to encourage involvement of the dad/partner? What can your partner do to help? What is their role in the postpartum journey? How can you best communicate your needs?

Please note that I use the term *partner* to designate the other parent, to encompass couples of all gender and sexual identities.

(I identify as a cis-female in a heterosexual relationship, so my stories will mention my husband, who is the father of my children.)

## MOM'S OVERWHELMING FEELINGS

New mothers often feel like they are the sole parent. This may be due to factors such as they are the only caregiver for the new baby, they are exclusively breastfeeding the baby, or they spend an extensive amount of time with the newborn during maternity leave while their partner must return to work. These feelings also may be due to social, cultural, or financial reasons. In any case, mothers often feel that they are alone in caring for their newborn once they arrive home.

Even though my husband was a 100% hands-on parent, doing what he could when he was home, I felt that all the baby's needs—feeding, changing, comforting, bathing, and sleeping—were on me. I didn't know where to put all this increased responsibility. I didn't know how to share it or communicate how I was feeling to my husband. As a pediatrician, I see mothers every day struggling with these same issues, juggling their duties as a mother while also managing their own feelings of stress and exhaustion. And although moms do the best they can, in these particular moments, they tend to feel guilty. We feel guilty, we feel bad, we feel resentful that the baby's needs fall upon us. And we feel guilty asking for help.

It is normal to feel as if we're not doing enough for our baby or not doing it well. It is normal to feel resentment that our spouse/partner may not be helping as much as we need or even that we have to ask (sometimes repeatedly) for help with household chores or baby care. Not only is it exhausting, but frankly it can be maddening.

What I know is this: *Mom guilt is very real.* Whether your child is 2 days, 2 months, 2 years, or 12 years old, mamas feel guilt; even if we are doing everything humanly possible to care for our child(ren), we still somehow feel that we are not doing it well enough. I am here to help you remove that unnecessary guilt.

> 66 During an office visit, a patient said to me, "I can count on one hand the number of hours I haven't been with the baby in the last 2 months. I just feel guilty and anxious because the baby is so small." 99

I am here to tell you, as a pediatrician and mother of 3, that caring for your newborn is *not* only your responsibility. You might be thinking, how can this be possible; I carried this child for 9 months, and I just gave birth, and now I am being sent home. I remember thinking, how are they sending me home with a brand-new human being? Where is my instruction guide? Of course I am responsible! So let me clarify. Of course, mom, you are responsible, but you are not the *only* one who is responsible. When my second child was born, my husband took both diapered children out for a walk in our neighborhood so I could get some rest. One of the neighbors exclaimed, "It's so great of you to babysit!" My husband was dumbfounded that anyone would think that caring for his children warranted congratulations. Both personally and professionally, I witness these things daily. Whether it's the father in my office who does not get up to change the baby's diaper as mom struggles to sit up after her cesarean delivery or the mother who is nursing while trying to juggle bedtime for her toddler because her husband is tired after work. The stories are endless. Again, although there may be societal, cultural, and familial factors at play, that does not mean this behavior is acceptable or has to continue. What I used to tell people who were worried about my husband when I was traveling to speak at a conference is that the last time I checked, he supplied 50% of the DNA for these children and is just as responsible for caring for them.

From the beginning, fathers/partners can and should be encouraged to interact with their newborn right after birth. Things such as bathing and diapering demonstrations in the hospital have led father to become more engaged right from the start. Fathers can also participate in feeding by supporting the breastfeeding mother or feed the baby once the baby is taking a bottle. In fact, the research shows that fathers do indeed want to be involved but are often unsure on how to be involved. Fathers may feel that the mother has all the answers and is confident in caring for the newborn while the father may feel inadequate. Starting with the knowledge that fathers/partners want to be involved can be help-ful as you navigate how to balance some of the responsibility.

### Strategies

Let's start with some basic strategies for involving your partner/father/significant other and communicating this expectation effectively. First and foremost, you are tired. Ask your partner to snuggle with the baby and rock the baby before putting him or her to sleep in the bassinette or crib. I know for my husband, this quiet uninterrupted time was very special. After feeding the baby, I give her to my husband to burp and change. And, yes, I am here to tell you that dads can change diapers. In fact, my husband, who had never changed a diaper in his life did a nice job in the hospital while I was resting after my cesarean deliv-ery. And, yes, the diaper actually stayed on. The postpartum nurse also taught him how to wrap her in a receiving blanket. To this day, my husband can snug an infant better than most.

It is important for dad/partner to feel empowered, to feel just as capable of learning to care for the infant as you are. Remember when I said that your partner will do things differently? Not only is that 100% okay, but you need not to micromanage how they go about doing things. So many times, mothers tell me they feel overwhelmed but admit that they feel their spouse/partner should just know what needs to be done. Your partner cannot read your mind (even though you wish they could). Please com-municate your needs and expectations to your spouse/partner. Believe me, that will allow you to get on the same page.

Even for my mamas who are exclusively breastfeeding, their partners can and should be involved. They need this special bonding time with their baby too. Many times, the partner feels left out because the baby spends a great deal of time breastfeeding, especially during those first few weeks. After nursing, please give the baby to your partner. This allows the partner to spend time with the baby and gives you an opportunity to rest, shower, eat, or spend time with an older child. In my case, in which I solely pumped for my first child (more on that later), dad would feed the baby freshly pumped milk while I went to rinse the pump parts. For my nursing mothers, although this may not be possible in those initial few weeks while you establish your milk supply, partners can still be involved. When it's time to nurse, ask your partner to bring the baby to you so you don't have to get out of bed. This is especially important in those first few days after delivery, especially for those who have had a cesarean delivery. While you nurse, your partner can help with other things, such as spending time with older siblings, cleaning up, or throwing in a load of laundry. These may seem like small tasks, but they add up and often cause stress for new mothers. Fathers/partners can care for the newborn after they get home so that mothers can have some special time with the older sibling.

For my moms who are formula feeding, the dad/partner can wash the bottles, prepare the formula, and feed the baby. This is a great opportunity for you to rest or, if you are not feeling exhausted, complete other tasks.

Regardless of how your baby is being fed, that 2- to 3-hour period after one feeding and before the next is a good opportunity for your partner to spend some bonding time with the baby. I cannot overemphasize the importance of this stretch of time from the end of one feed until the start of the next feed. It may only be 2 hours or less in those early weeks, but this is the time for mom to rest. Although you may not fall into a deep sleep, which is fine, I need my mamas to rest. This rest is so important for your body to heal and your mind to rest. Discussing the importance of rest and time to recover with your partner/spouse early on is essential so your needs and expectations are defined. It will also lessen any feelings that you are doing everything on your own, which may cause resentment.

> ### Typical Partner Responses
> ### When a New Baby Arrives
>
> "I don't know what to do; all he does is nurse and I feel useless."
>
> "I'm not comfortable changing her, she is so tiny."
>
> "I don't know how to do that, and you'll just end up doing it over."

I know this may be difficult for some of you. Believe me, I completely understand. In my case, with my first baby, I felt that I needed to clean, do laundry, and finish those baby shower thank-you notes—basically do anything *but* rest. Regardless of whether the pressure comes from within us or from family members, this is not what new mothers should be doing. This added pressure, whether its origin is societal, familial, cultural, or personal, is not OK, and it is definitely not conducive to your physical and mental postpartum health. Sleep and rest are essential, especially in those early weeks and months.

Your partner may feel as if he or she can't help you care for the baby, but this is 100% untrue. Sometimes, it may be up to you, as the mother, to guide your partner on how they can be involved while helping you get the rest you need. Remember, it's important for your partner to have time with the new baby. Your partner wants to cuddle and smell the newborn's head too. Although those early weeks are chaotic (at least they were in our house), have that conversation with your partner. Remember, no one is a mind reader, so it's OK to tell your partner what you need from them. But they need to tell you how they are feeling too. Moms, remember it is important for you not to micromanage the time between your newborn and spouse/partner. Fathers/partners need the time and freedom to develop their own relationship with the baby, and often this role will complement what mothers do for their baby. Fathers' interaction with the baby will not be identical to mothers', and that is okay. It is not for you to dictate or criticize. Give your spouse/partner the space and opportunity to build their own unique relationship with the baby. This will allow your spouse/partner to feel confident and secure as a parent. And trust me, doing this early on in the fourth trimester will pay off down the road.

## *How to Express Your Need for Help*

How can you do this? Of course, it will depend in part on your style of communication, but being direct is key. Remember, humans can't read minds, and that includes your spouse or partner. You may feel uncomfortable asking for help because you think you should be able to handle it all. Or there might be a perception that the person who works outside the home is working harder than you and should not be expected to help with the baby and other household tasks. Again, the postpartum plan (Chapter 4) will help with many of these concerns because you have already outlined and planned for many of the issues that may be occurring at this moment. But one important thing to remember, what you are going through, mama, is not something your spouse or partner will understand. The pregnancy, birth/delivery, and postpartum physical and mental changes, well, those are unique to you, the mother. But it is important to communicate your needs, frustrations, and concerns to your partner before they build up, causing unnecessary resentment.

It is important to keep in mind that fathers can also develop postpartum depression and may require support. Symptoms may present differently; instead of sadness, they may present as anger or irritability and even may undermine the mother's care of the baby, including breastfeeding. As discussed in Chapter 4, fathers may also need help and should be encouraged to seek counseling. Again, your baby's pediatrician/pediatric healthcare provider is a good resource to ask for help.

## *Older Siblings*

In addition to tackling and sharing domestic tasks, such as laundry, washing dishes, cooking meals, and paying bills, moms and dads need to carve out some special time for any older siblings. While mom is feeding and/or resting, this is a good time for the partner to take care of and play with the older children. Remember, a new baby is an adjustment for the older children too, regardless of their ages, so while life at home may not be the same, it is important to maintain some of their normal activities and schedules. Also, consider scheduling some special activities or outings during which the attention is solely on the siblings.

I am frequently helping new moms juggle the activities of multiple children. I know for me, it was very difficult to nurse and manage a colicky newborn without feeling guilty that I was neglecting my toddler. Once you are done nursing or if your partner is bottle feeding the newborn, this is a great time to be with your older child(ren). Whether it's playing a game, watching a video while lying in bed together, reading a book, or going for a walk, it's the quality of the time together, not the quantity that is important. It may be tempting to multitask while your baby sleeps, but it is so important to give your undivided attention to the older sibling. So put away your phone, turn off the TV, and don't worry about unloading the dishwasher. So, no, you don't have to take them to the park or an indoor play space, which will only exhaust you. Enjoy that cuddle time with your other children too.

### Important Tips for Older Siblings

Explain what it will be like when the new baby arrives. This can be done through play, conversations, or books.

When the new baby arrives, have someone bring your older child to the hospital to meet and cuddle the new baby. Make sure to check your hospitals rules and regulations for visitors during this time.

Give the older sibling a special gift from the baby.

Carve out time for just you and your older child(ren), doing something special for him or her.

One important point is for you, mom, to get *restful* rest. You're probably thinking, what does that even mean; rest is rest. Well, no, all rest is not equal. Let me give you an example: You lie down but can hear the baby cooing and/or the toddler yelling in another room. I don't know about other moms, but if I heard my baby crying or a child yelling, I was definitely not going to get any rest. This is what I tell my dads/partners: Take the baby (along with older siblings) outside for a walk. I am a huge fan of baby carriers. My husband absolutely loved having the baby snuggled into his chest while his hands were free to push a stroller, hold the toddler's hand, or push a swing. Plus, newborns love that closeness and will fall asleep with that movement. Just be sure you are using the carrier correctly with proper placement of the newborn's body and head.

## IMPORTANCE OF EATING AND DRINKING

Between baby duties and household tasks, many women often forget to feed themselves. And while nutrition and hydration are important for all moms, they are especially important for breastfeeding mothers to maintain their milk supply (see Chapter 7). When I was at home with my first-born, I was pumping around the clock, feeding her pumped milk, cleaning pump parts, and doing laundry and everything else that needed to be done. You know what I ate while I pumped? A candy bar or something equally nonnutritious that I could grab with one hand. Yes, I am being totally serious.

For mamas who are concerned about diet, nutrition, and weight loss, I will cover those topics (and more) in Chapter 8.

Back to eating. We often forget, put it off, or try to sustain ourselves through various drinks, but doing so will make you feel tired and really hungry, may tank your breast milk supply, and overall will just not be helpful as you recover from childbirth. So what can you do? I'll tell you what I tell mothers in my practice every single day: When the baby eats, so do you. That's easy to remember, right?

Here are some easy things that dad/partner/significant other can do to be involved in caring for you *and* the baby:

- Hydration: Fill up a big water bottle for mama to drink all day. I love ice water, the colder the better. And I'm not talking about one of those plastic bottles. I suggest buying an insulated metal water bottle from your favorite store. (It's better for the environment too!) Keep filling it up all day (and night).

- Meals: Dad can prepare protein-rich meals if he is fortunate to have family leave. But I tell my parents that before he leaves for work or after he gets home, preparing a large meal that mom can eat while he cares for the newborn is important.

- The dad/mom (or insert name here) basket: After a friend mentioned this to me years ago, I now tell all my parents to do this. Keep a basket (or any container) next to your bed that dad/partner can keep filled with nutritious snacks for mom to grab with one hand while nursing or bottle feeding the baby. Be sure these snacks are healthy and rich in protein.

Of course, preparing a smoothie or protein shake that day or the night before is a great way to keep mom hydrated while making sure she gets the nutrition and protein she needs. Again, another great way to involve your partner.

## MOMS LEARN TO LET GO

I'd like to address an issue that I feel many mothers struggle with: letting go. Whether it's changing a diaper, preparing a bottle, doing laundry, or going grocery shopping, it is important for you relinquish those responsibilities in the early weeks and months. You also have to be OK with how dad/partner performs these tasks. And, yes, your partner will do them differently than you do them.

I'm not going to lie; as a physician-mommy and the oldest child in my family, I am and have always been a type A personality. I do well with order and lists. I don't think I am alone in this feeling that things have to be done in a certain way for them to be done the "right way." When I talk with fellow mothers, whether they are friends, colleagues, or new mothers in my practice, I always remind them that their partner will do things differently, and that is OK. Mama, you have just got to let that stuff go. And believe me, this is a good skill to have, not just for you and your partner, but for the rest of your household. So no judgment, OK?

To this day, with 3 teenagers in our house, my husband takes a really long time grocery shopping, no I mean really long. But guess what? That's what works for him, and because he's cooking, he is allowed to be particular about the groceries. Remember, as your child(ren) get older, it's important for everyone in the house to have their own responsibilities and age-appropriate chores. But that's a whole other book!

The important thing is for your partner to be involved in taking care of baby, you, your older children, and the household. Remember, this is a team sport and you are not supposed to do it all. Becoming overly stressed and utterly exhausted is not going to help you or your baby. So talk with your partner, tell him or her what you need during this postpartum period. Do not feel guilty about it. As your baby grows and your family changes, so will your needs, and that's 100% normal. I encourage you to communicate with your partner so he or she will know how to help. Whether that means feeding the baby, cleaning the house, making sure you are nourished, or just taking the kids out of the house so you can get a restful sleep, this division of labor is essential for your mental and physical health and well-being.

Remember my mantra: *Happy and healthy mama equals happy and healthy baby.*

CHAPTER 6

# Visitors/Boundaries

**VISITOR**/noun /ˈvizidər/: a person visiting a person or place

> ❝ I remember feeling so overwhelmed when visitors made up of neighbors, friends, and family would call on weekends to want to come and see the baby. I was by myself all week and my husband was only home on the weekends. I was trying to balance our time as a family too. I felt so frustrated trying to find appropriate clothes that still fit me. Some family members became offended when I asked them to wash their hands. It was just so exhausting. I felt like I had to entertain when all I wanted to do was sleep while others held the baby. ❞

*W*hen I became a new mom, saying that I felt overwhelmed was an understatement, to say the least. Trying to nurse (which I couldn't), pumping every 3 hours, walking around like a zombie on very little sleep, attempting to complete housework and actually eat, well, it was all just so exhausting. Honestly, the last thing I wanted to do was get out of my comfortable large t-shirt and sweatpants, wash my hair, and make myself look presentable to friends and family who wanted to visit the baby.

As part of Indian culture, just like many cultures around the world, it is common for family and friends to come over to see the newborn and give their blessings. Although I appreciated this, it was just too much for me. There was no way I could find a top that would fit over my huge breasts filled with milk. And, honestly, if there were male relatives and friends in the room, nursing in front of visitors was extremely uncomfortable. There were also cultural nuances I had to respect, but also the timing of the feeds and baby's naps were completely screwed up depending on what time visitors decided to drop by. It was all so overwhelming. And while it is important for both parents to set boundaries, I think it is difficult to say no to people who want to visit the baby. Other moms have told me that when they left the room to breastfeed, family and friends would ask them where they were going or say, "Didn't he just eat?" Even writing this down brings back all those stressful feelings.

Germs are a valid concern of new mamas. As a pediatrician, I was super anxious about having a bunch of people holding and breathing on my baby. Like most new moms, I didn't want my baby exposed to germs and possible illness. And as a pediatrician, I knew what tests and examinations my newborn would have to endure if she developed a fever. It wasn't as simple as giving her acetaminophen and letting her sleep. Don't hesitate to ask all visitors to wash their hands before touching or holding your newborn. You and your partner should set your rules and let all your visitors know.

## TAKING, SHARING, AND POSTING PHOTOS

Another important issue to consider is sharing of photos. Your visitors will not only want to hold the new bundle of joy, but their smartphones are always a short reach away. While digital photography had begun when my kids were babies, there were no smartphones like there are now. As soon as a picture is taken, it can get sent, shared, and posted within seconds. You won't even see the flashbulb go off, but before you sit down, you can see your baby's cute photo on Facebook.

You and your partner need to be clear with visitors regarding your house rules. It is OK to tell your friend, neighbor, or cousin that certain days and times work better than others. Don't hesitate to reach out to visitors and ask them to delay their visit until you feel better and are more rested. You might also ask visitors to wait a few weeks before coming into your home, although you will continue to have to take precautions when they are around the newborn.

Instruct anyone who comes into your home to wash their hands before reaching for the baby. Also, depending on how comfortable you and your partner feel, do not hesitate to tell grandma or your best friend that they are not to post pictures of your newborn until you give the green light.

## LET'S TALK ABOUT BOUNDARIES

Boundaries are your limits. But as women and mothers, we sometimes have difficulty enforcing limits. We feel bad. We may feel as though we are disappointing others. And when we bring our newborn home, the expectation is that anyone and everyone should be able to visit and see the baby. Of course, we need to keep in mind familial and cultural expectations, but I want you to remember that as a mother with a newborn, you can impose limits. It is OK to say no. It may not be easy (it never was for me until baby No. 3), but it needs to be done. In addition, it is essential that you and your spouse/partner are on the same page because you will need support, and your partner may need to step in to enforce those boundaries.

Deciding how you and your partner want to handle visitors is best done before the delivery. A good time to discuss this is during the last trimester of your pregnancy while formulating your postpartum plan. Of course, the specifics may change after you come home with the baby, but having a game plan in place for how to handle visit requests will be extremely helpful.

Many new moms feel as though they are alone in this. I hope that in this chapter you can find strategies to help manage visitors, friends, and family once you return home with your newborn. However, it's important to remember that this is not solely your responsibility. Your husband/significant other/partner must take responsibility for helping to set boundaries, especially during those early days. As I address in Chapter 4, I encourage you and your partner to do the bulk of this planning during the pregnancy because this will help guide your decisions after the baby is born.

## TALK TOGETHER ABOUT YOUR PLAN AT ALL STAGES

When thinking about who you want to help you, be sure to consider all stages: pregnancy, at the birth, and after delivery.

### Postpartum Help

Who will be with you when you come home from the hospital with your newborn? For some families, this may be your mother, while for others this may be your mother-in-law. Many factors, including family and cultural reasons, may impact your decisions. However, I want to remind you of something important. In those early days, it is important to have a person or persons who will be helpful in caring not just for the baby but for you as well. Regardless of your familial or cultural expectations, if a situation doesn't help you rest and heal, then you can choose to say no. I tell my mamas all the time that it does not matter how your mom, your mother-in-law, or other family members managed their postpartum periods. This is about *you*. And only you are in charge of your postpartum journey, including who will be there to help you in the early days and weeks.

Once you come home, whether you are breastfeeding or formula feeding, you will be sleep-deprived. You will also be recovering from giving birth. Remember mama, you just grew and nourished a human being, and after 9 months you did some hard physical labor to bring this baby into the world. Often, we forget the physical aspect of giving birth and the toll it has taken on our bodies. Therefore, whoever you choose to be with you in the early postpartum days will also be there to take care of you.

Please be sure that you and your partner are on the same page regarding the role this person or persons will have. This should be part of your early conversations. Often, mothers aren't always the best at articulating what they need. This was definitely me! I was sleep-deprived, sore from my cesarean delivery, and just in a general fog. I thought I could and should do most of the work instead of asking for help. Who else has trouble asking for help?

### *Learn to Ask Your Guests for Help*
I know it can be difficult to ask "guests" to do what seem like chores, but this is what you and baby need during this time. And that is OK. Remember, your family and friends want to help you. I still recall when my friend with whom I did my pediatric residency came over to my apartment on a weekday afternoon. She literally sat in my living room, watched TV, and held and fed the baby. Why did she come over? So I could get my hair cut, colored, and styled. I still remember; it was a glorious afternoon, all to myself and all for me.

You need to take time for yourself during the day. As women and as mothers, we often want to make sure that everyone else is doing OK and almost feel as if we need to entertain those who have come into our home. In many cultures and families, like my own, there is a definite expectation to entertain and feed guests. But again, setting expectations before the baby arrives will make a world of difference in those early postpartum days and weeks.

## Define Family Roles Early On

Family:

Prior to the arrival of your family, be sure to define their specific roles:

- Preparing and cooking family meals
- Going grocery shopping
- Helping to clean the house and doing laundry
- Caring for older siblings
- Driving older kids to and from school

Friends:

For your friends who reach out and ask what they can do to help, here are some ideas to consider:

- Drive you and your baby to a doctor appointment
- Stop by to throw in a quick load of laundry
- Bring a meal that you can throw in the oven
- Take your older children to the park so you can nap
- Ask the friend to stop over during the day so you can shower and wash your hair
- Wash the baby bottles and nipples
- Fill up or empty the dishwasher
- Ask the friend to stop over so you can nap

Each family is different. For many of my friends who immigrated to this country, various family members came at different times depending on the postpartum stage. Initially, the mother's parents came, and then as the baby grew older, the father's parents came. Although their roles will differ, if this arrangement works for your family, it is important to have both sets of grandparents help out. Grandma can physically care for baby and mama, while grandpa can play with the older children or do household chores or other needed tasks. It is OK to ask visitors, regardless of their familial role or gender, to help. When long-term visitors come to your home in the early postpartum weeks, it is not a hotel or a vacation for them. They are not there to be entertained, waited on, or fed 3 meals a day. Set that expectation up front so you and your partner are on the same page. If they are not able to help you in ways in which you need to be helped, then they probably shouldn't be at your home during the early postpartum period. Talking about expectations up front will help to reduce stress after the baby arrives. Family members can visit later on when you're ready. And that is OK. I promise.

## WHAT ABOUT THOSE WHO WANT TO STOP BY?

We have many good friends, colleagues, and neighbors who are always excited to meet the new baby. I too become excited to check on mama and meet the newborn, but I have to stop and remind myself that those early days are not for me to just drop by. Again, articulating your needs as a new mother is so important. Doing so will not only get everyone on the same page, but it will also help to lessen your frustration.

Your close friends and other mothers will probably know exactly what you need, which is great! Be sure to tell them what food to bring you or when to pick you up for a night out. Whether it's having a meal train sign-up, putting a do-not-disturb sign on your front door, or texting another mom to pick up your toddler for a play date, this is a great way to let people know what you need and, more importantly, what will help you and your family. Being clear about what you need at that particular time will also be appreciated by your family and friends so they don't have to guess.

As you wrote in your postpartum plan, remember to prepare that list of friends or neighbors you can reach out to when you need a break. This will be especially important if and when your partner returns to work and you are home alone with your baby. Having a list of friends who are available, while taking into account their varying schedules, is essential. When you need to take a nap or a shower, who will be your person(s) to contact?

When your newborn needs a well-child (health supervision) visit, whom will you call? There will also be times when you just want to have another adult to talk to or a friend to hang out with while you're home all day. Who will that person be?

It may seem silly to have a call list, but I wish that I had done this years ago. When I was struggling with mastitis and called a friend to come help me because my husband had to leave for work, I remember how sad and frustrated I was when she said she couldn't come over. I felt so dejected, so sad. I honestly didn't feel like asking anyone else for help, and I didn't. I just pushed through with body aches, chills, and fever while continuing to pump and take care of a newborn.

Those who want to stop by to see the baby need to work around mom's sleep schedule too. Period. Your rest comes first, mama. Although a guest can drop by and peek into the crib of a sleeping newborn, this won't work for a mother who needs her own sleep. If a particular day or time doesn't work, you and/or your partner need to be clear about that. The worst times for me were when people wanted to stop by after work. Trying to handle a toddler, nurse a newborn, and take a shower while being in my pajamas all day—not to mention getting some sort of dinner ready—well, no, that is not a good time. Back then, I wish someone had told me that it was okay to just say no without being fearful of offending someone. And when you are too tired or just don't want to make those decisions, your partner needs to step in. You are not in this alone, mama.

## WHAT TO DO ABOUT SICK VISITORS

Another important issue is the health and safety of your baby. When I see newborns in my office, I always discuss illness and fever. The No. 1 take-home point is that people who are ill, have a cough, cold, fever, or stomach flu should not come over to see the new baby. Not even a family member or grandparent. While a fever and viral illness do not adversely affect older children or adults, they *can* severely impact a newborn. A fever in a newborn is defined as a temperature of 100.4°F (38°C) or higher. A baby with a fever undergoes blood, urine, and other invasive tests. Thus, do not be afraid to establish rules for your visitors. And I'll tell you what I tell my moms: If they get upset, you can blame me, your friendly neighborhood pediatrician.

## SET BOUNDARIES

I know I have given you and your partner a lot to think about and digest. But one thing you need to remember: Please set your boundaries early. Believe me, speaking as a mama, doing so will not only benefit you and your newborn in that early postpartum period, but you will see those benefits within your entire family structure. As women, we are often taught to please others and accept things as they are. Well, that mindset has to change. It may not be easy, but telling your partner, family, and friends what you need during those early postpartum days is so import- ant for you and your baby. You need to heal. You need to rest. You need to regain your strength. Surround yourself with those who will allow you to do these things.

What do I always say? *Happy and healthy mama equals happy and healthy baby.*

CHAPTER 7

# Infant Nutrition

NUTRITION/noun /n(y)ooˈtriSH(ə)n/: the process of providing or obtaining the food necessary for health and growth

As a pediatrician, I inform each mom and family about the benefits of breastfeeding. However, my intent is not to make any mama feel bad if she is not exclusively breastfeeding or she decided to feed her baby formula. However, as a doctor, it is my responsibility to give new moms realistic advice while providing the facts. This is important because based on what others tell you, what you read on social media, or what you may perceive, there is no *right way* to feed your baby. I don't want any of you to feel that you are a *bad mom* because you chose differently from your mother, your sister, or your friend. Every mom, every baby, and every situation is different.

I struggled with breastfeeding for all 3 of my children, and, yes, they all received formula during the first year after birth. But many times, new mamas struggle with breastfeeding and give up, then later feel guilty because they received advice, read something completely incorrect online, or just didn't receive the support they needed in those early days. That is why I want to clear up this confusion and give you the facts. Because of my own breastfeeding struggles, coupled with mommy guilt, I am a breastfeeding medicine specialist who helps moms and babies to breastfeed—based on what mom's goals are. My hope is that the advice I have been giving to my mamas in practice for years will help many of you. I do this so other moms do not have to struggle like I did. Each time, when I introduce myself to a mama-baby pair, I tell the mother that my struggles brought me here in the hopes that I can help them. And most, if not all, appreciate that I struggled and that, no, it wasn't perfect.

> 66 Just because it's natural doesn't mean it's easy. 99

If you don't remember anything else from this chapter, remember this quote. I remember when I struggled with breastfeeding, I kept thinking, What is wrong with me and my boobs? I'm doing this all wrong! It was especially frustrating because I had friends and colleagues who nursed their babies without any issues. However, just because you have breasts does not mean it is easy. I am here to tell you it most definitely is *not*. Breastfeeding can be difficult. But with the right support and correct advice, it can be done, making it an enjoyable bonding experience for you and your baby.

## BENEFITS OF BREASTFEEDING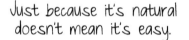

Although I am not going to belabor the benefits of breastfeeding, I also don't want to assume that everyone reading this (or your spouse/partner/family members) is aware. Breastfeeding has been shown to lower the risk of asthma (even if there is a smoker in your house), allergies, ear infections, pneumonia, diabetes, and gastrointestinal illnesses in children. Many of you may already know these facts, but I have found throughout the years that many women (and their support system) are unaware of the numerous benefits for mom. Breastfeeding reduces the risk of heart disease, high blood pressure, diabetes, and breast and ovarian cancer. And guess what? You don't have to exclusively breastfeed to experience these benefits. For instance, if you breastfed your first baby for 4 months, then your second baby for 6 months, those 10 months add up to decrease your risk of breast cancer.

After taking all the medical evidence into account, this is what I tell every single one of my mothers: *Some breastfeeding is better than none.* So if you are a mom who breastfed for a month, 6 months, or a year, you and the baby will receive those benefits.

## LET'S START AT THE BEGINNING

Don't worry, this isn't a history lesson, though you will learn some anatomical terms. During pregnancy, there is a rapid growth of the components of the system that will help initiate, continue, and deliver breast milk to your baby. The breast is supplied by various nerves, blood vessels, and the lymphatic system, which is important for various reasons. For women who have had breast surgery, such as breast implants or a breast reduction, depending on the surgery and the nerves and vessels that may have been affected, breast milk production might be impacted. Many new mamas in my office were never told that their surgery could affect their nursing goals. This is not to say that you won't be able to breastfeed, but prior surgery may affect supply, and some mothers may have to supplement. If you have had any breast surgery, please talk to your surgeon about how this may affect breastfeeding.

Another important thing to understand is that breastfeeding is *not* nipple feeding. Although some may have difficulty nursing because of their nipple and areola, having flat or inverted nipples is not a reason for you to be unable to breastfeed. In fact, most women have pain with nursing because babies tend to have a shallow latch, causing them to solely attach to and suck on the nipple. Ouch! Remember those nerves I was talking about? The nerve endings converge on your nipple. So I want your baby to open wide to take not only the nipple but part of the areola into the mouth too.

Women have breasts that come in all sizes, which is what makes each and every one of you beautifully unique. But your breast size does not determine how much milk you will make. In fact, there is no correlation between your breast growth during pregnancy and your milk production in that first month. No matter what your cup size is, your breasts will (and should) grow during pregnancy. However, your breast size will determine capacity, that is, women with smaller breasts will have their breasts emptied faster than a woman with larger breasts because larger breasts will be able to hold more milk. However, your breast size will not limit how much milk you can and will produce for your baby, so I don't want my mamas with A and B cups to stress about this.

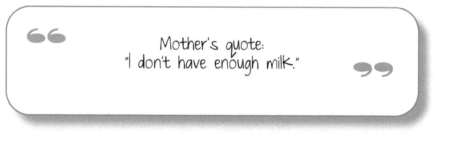

66

Mother's quote:
"I don't have enough milk."

99

I cannot tell you how many times I have heard this statement throughout my career from moms who feel frustrated. But medically speaking, true lactation failure occurs in less than 5% of women. Most of the time, when mamas see a slowdown in their milk production, they tell me they have "dried up." However, in all likelihood, this is due to a disruption in the supply-demand chain.

During pregnancy, your breast is beginning to form and synthesize those early pathways and milk components. Soon after delivery, your breast will start to produce milk and your breasts will begin to feel full. Some people refer to this as their milk "coming in." Generally speaking, it was thought that most women will feel this fullness within 2 to 4 days after giving birth. This period is referred to as *lactogenesis II.* However, based on various anatomical, physiologic, and hormonal effects, this is not the case for every woman.

## Maternal Conditions That May Cause a Delay in Lactogenesis II

- Obesity
- Cesarean delivery
- Diabetes
- Hypothyroidism
- Stress
- Complications during delivery

Unfortunately, at least in the United States, most moms are discharged from the hospital within 2 to 3 days after delivery, so this initial let-down may occur when mom is at home. This may exacerbate feelings of anxiety, especially because there is little support once you leave the hospital. I encourage you, mama, to ask to be seen by a lactation consultant before you and your baby are discharged. You can ask her any questions you may have, as well as receive information about outpatient support.

*Colostrum* is the initial milk that will be available almost immediately. After delivery, even after a cesarean delivery, we recommend putting the baby to your breast within the first hour, also known as the "golden hour." Let your baby suckle at your nipple. This will help stimulate your milk production. After that first hour, your newborn will become very drowsy and less likely to want to nurse. So, before your delivery, depending on the hospital, be sure to advocate for your baby and yourself so you can have immediate skin-to-skin contact with your newborn. Of course, this may not happen if there are any medical concerns for mom or baby.

When I delivered my second child, the doctor explained to me that his temperature was dropping. So instead of placing him on my chest, which is the ultimate baby warmer, they put him in an incubator/warmer. Then I experienced great difficulty getting him to nurse because he was so drowsy. So please, advocate for yourself or, better yet, tell your spouse (or whomever will be in the delivery room or operating room with you) to advocate *for* you. I gave my husband specific instructions, which I found helpful, not just for me and the baby, but for him too because he knew exactly what I needed him to do once the baby was delivered. Remember, your significant other is probably feeling just as joyful as you are once your baby arrives. Giving clear-cut instructions usually is welcomed by your partner.

That initial colostrum you produce in the first few days is sufficient for your baby. I always tell my moms that the newborn's stomach is the size of his or her fist.

Since your newborn's stomach is so small, there's no need to feed 2 or 3 ounces in the first few days. The small amount of colostrum your body makes is just the right amount for your newborn. The key is to put your baby to your breast to stimulate that nipple *every single time* your newborn is hungry. That nipple stimulation is a signal to your brain to continue to produce colostrum, which later on will turn into mature milk. For my mamas who may be having difficulty nursing, who may not want to nurse, or who may be separated from their baby, this can also be done

## The Average Size of a Newborn's Stomach

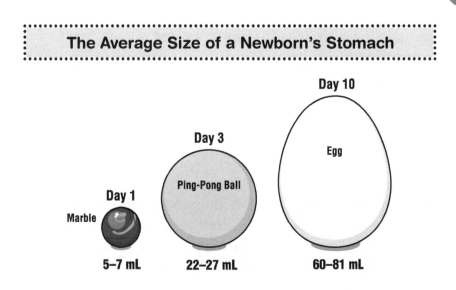

Day 10

Egg

Day 3

Ping-Pong Ball

Day 1

Marble

5–7 mL          22–27 mL          60–81 mL

with a pump. It may be a bit more difficult because colostrum is thicker than mature milk and there will be smaller amounts, but do not stress. You are not supposed to see ounces of milk flowing through that pump in the early days. Again, this is a great time to ask to be seen by a lactation consultant so you can ask her about colostrum, nursing, and even pumping.

### Colostrum

Colostrum is also known as baby's first immunization because it is filled with many antibodies and nutrients that can help fight off infection and disease. However, because it looks quite different from mature milk, in some cultures, colostrum is viewed as dirty and is discarded. This denial of colostrum is practiced across the globe in various Asian, African, and Latin American countries.

## Supply and Demand

After that initial automatic production of breast milk, the only way to continue producing milk is to remove it from your breast. Yes, ladies, use it or lose it. Those first few weeks are *so* important, not only to start building up your supply but also to maintain it, which is fueled by milk removal.

A woman's body is pretty amazing. As long as milk continues to be removed from the breast, the milk production, also known as *lactogenesis*, will continue. Your newborn stimulates your nipple, which will cause let-down, and as your baby continues to nurse, this milk removal will guarantee continued production. This process is the same for my pumping mamas who will be expressing, essentially removing, breast milk with a pump. What *will* slow down your breast milk production and put you at risk for complete cessation is ineffective or infrequent nursing or expressing. There is this amazing physiologic mechanism called a negative feedback loop that signals to your brain when breast milk production needs to speed up (your breasts are emptying) or slow down (your breasts are full).

Breast milk is rather amazing. It changes during the feed, throughout the day, and as the baby grows. Seriously, pretty cool right? The beginning of the feed is called the *foremilk*, while the milk at the end of the feed is called *hindmilk*. The foremilk is starchy and looks very thin while the hindmilk contains the fat your baby needs for brain development, to feel full, and to gain weight. Basically, what I tell my moms is that breast milk starts with skim milk and ends with ice cream.

### Empty One Breast

The key is to fully empty 1 breast while nursing. I do not want you to block feed, which is 5 or 10 minutes on 1 breast and then 5 or 10 minutes on the other breast. This will not fully empty your breasts, which can adversely affect your supply, but it also will not allow your baby to feel full and satisfied because he or she will only be receiving the foremilk, the starchier component. So here's the trick. When your baby is hungry (don't wait more than 3 hours), put your baby on the breast. Fully empty that breast. When it starts emptying, you will definitely feel the difference; I call the emptier one a deflated balloon. The baby will probably nurse for a maximum of 15 to 20 minutes on that breast. Do *not* allow your baby to hang out on 1 breast for 40 minutes and use you as a pacifier (yes, I see that all the time!). Remove your baby from that breast, burp the baby, and if the baby is still hungry, offer the second breast. In those early days, your newborn will likely take only 1 breast because their stomachs are small. (See The Average Size of a Newborn's Stomach on page 67.)

Because you are tired and sleep deprived, I want you to put one of those elastic hair ties around the wrist of the side you are going to start nursing on after the baby wakes up. If you just completed the left breast, put your hair tie on the right wrist so it will remind you to start the baby on the right side for the next feed. I know many things are sold on the market, but you really only need a generic elastic hair tie. And for my type A mamas, while you may thrive on schedules and apps, please do not make more work for yourselves. Monitoring how much your baby urinates and stools is important. While urine output is a good indicator of the baby's hydration status, the amount of stool is a more sensitive indicator of how many calories your baby is getting. Your newborn should have at least 1 to 2 bowel movements per day. Monitoring output while your pediatrician monitors your baby's weight gain will hopefully reassure you that you and your breast milk are doing just fine. While your baby is napping until the next feed in 2 to 3 hours, I need you to lie down and rest. No cleaning, no cooking, no writing thank-you cards for the baby shower gifts.

Lie down and rest.

Doctor's orders.

If you skip a nursing session, for instance if you are sleeping or taking your toddler to school or want to meet up with a friend or your mom is going to give the baby a bottle, just remember that you will have to remove that milk from your breast or risk a dip in your supply. Remember to always empty your breasts, whether this is through nursing, expression, or pumping approximately 8 to 12 times per day.

## Hand Expression

I'll be honest, I never heard the term *hand expression* when I was having babies. Although I did do something similar, I wasn't taught as a mom or trained in this as a pediatrician. Hand expression is important for many reasons. It can help stimulate your breasts when you are separated from your baby. It can also relieve pressure from engorged breasts. Additionally, it is a way to increase your supply and provide milk for your baby. And for my mamas with overactive let-down, this is a better way to help express than initial let-down to prevent your baby from gagging. My favorite videos showing this technique are from Stanford University (https://med.stanford.edu/ newborns/professional-education/breastfeeding/hand-expressing-milk.html), but others are available too. Again, this is a great question for the lactation consultant, who can show you how to do this before you leave the hospital.

What does this mean for you mama, practically speaking? When the baby is hungry, you should put your baby to the breast to feed. There is no schedule. I repeat, there is *no* schedule. I don't want you looking at a clock and giving your baby a pacifier to keep him or her calm while waiting for that 3-hour mark to feed your baby. If someone tells you that or you read that somewhere, he or she is wrong. Plain and simple.

### How Often to Feed

You will be feeding a healthy full-term newborn approximately every 1 to 3 hours. While every newborn is different, I give general guidelines to mothers encouraging them to feed their baby when they are hungry; there is no schedule during those early days and weeks. And as a general rule, especially in those early days, breastfed babies should not go more than 3 to 4 hours without feeding. And regardless of when they are feeding, newborns should not be sleeping through the night. Most of the time, breastfed babies poop more because breast milk is more easily digested than formula. I remember that my son would poop while nursing! I let him finish nursing and then, of course, changed the diaper before putting him down in his bassinette. Your baby's weight will be monitored closely by the pediatrician. Generally speaking, babies can lose 8% of their birth weight in those early days; however, once your milk production is abundant, your newborn should not continue to lose weight. While we generally give newborns 10 days to regain their birth weight, I monitor breastfeeding mamas more frequently because breastfed babies tend to gain weight at a slower rate than formula-fed babies. Again, please consult your pediatrician about any questions or concerns you have. I tell my mamas emphatically that they will be seeing me a lot in those first few weeks.

Another important factor to consider is jaundice, also known as hyperbilirubinemia. Jaundice is a common occurrence that generally is corrected with more frequent feeding. However, depending on the growth of the baby as well as the extent of the jaundice, your pediatrician may make some suggestions so the baby is growing adequately. For my exclusively breastfeeding mamas, if your pediatrician recommends some formula supple- mentation, do not feel defeated or feel that something is wrong with you and your breast milk. Nothing could be further from the truth. Although there are medical recommendations regarding when and how much to supplement, most of the time this is just a temporary measure.

## Jaundice

What is jaundice? Many babies have a slight yellow discoloration of their skin and eyes. This occurs because of an excess amount of bilirubin, which is a pigment in red blood cells. Jaundice develops because the baby's liver isn't mature enough to get rid of the excess bilirubin in the blood stream. In most babies, this is normal physiology, but some babies may have an underlying disease. Your baby's bilirubin levels will be checked before your baby leaves the hospital and likely will be rechecked at your pediatrician's office.

## Breastfeeding Issues

What if you want to provide breast milk to your baby but have difficulty nursing or just don't want to nurse. And that is fine. Many mothers in my practice, for their own personal reasons, do not want to nurse. In fact, with my first child, because of the lack of support and my lack of knowledge, I was never able to nurse. After crying and feeling frustrated that first week, I just decided that I would pump. And pump I did for 9 straight months. Although it is not easy, it can be done. But if you do decide to solely pump, the same rules apply. You must fully empty your breasts every 3 hours during the first few weeks to maintain and increase your supply.

Whether your baby is suckling at your nipple or you are using a breast pump, some mamas may feel that *let-down reflex*, almost like a tingling sensation. However, don't be panicked if you don't experience this sensation, as not all mothers feel this but clearly have let-down. This is a negative mechanical pressure generated

### What Is Dysphoric Milk Ejection Reflex (D-MER)?

You may feel sad, unhappy, or panicky right before your breasts let-down milk.

This should only last for a few minutes.

It is thought to be brought on by various hormones that get activated while breastfeeding.

It may be so distressing to some mothers that they don't feel like breastfeeding.

Just know that you are not doing anything wrong. The feeling will pass, so don't give up on your breastfeeding goals.

Strategies to help minimize the symptoms of D-MER include surrounding yourself with support, practicing mindfulness, and increasing skin-to-skin contact with your baby.

If feelings of sadness or worry persist, please speak to your obstetrician.

to release oxytocin—also known as the love hormone—that will start the flow of milk. Many of you may feel that tingling sensation when it starts. Some of you may experience let-down when you are separated from your baby but think of your baby or even hear the cry of another baby. This is where breast pads come in handy to prevent leakage onto your shirt. Let-down can be inhibited by fear, pain, embarrassment, and anxiety. So being forced

| Human Milk Storage Guidelines | | | |
|---|---|---|---|
| **Type of Breast Milk** | **Storage Location and Temperatures** | | |
| | Countertop 77°F (25°C) or colder (room temperature) | Refrigerator 40°F (4°C) | Freezer 0°F (-18°C) or colder |
| **Freshly Expressed or Pumped** | Up to **4 Hours** | Up to **4 Days** | Within **6 months** is best<br>Up to **12 months** is acceptable |
| **Thawed, Previously Frozen** | **1–2 Hours** | Up to **1 Day** (24 hours) | *Never* refreeze human milk after it has been thawed |
| **Leftover From a Feeding** (baby did not finish the bottle) | Use within **2 hours** after the baby is finished feeding | | |

https://www.cdc.gov/breastfeeding/recommendations/handling_breastmilk.htm

to pump in a bathroom stall or feeling shamed to nurse in public may be situations in which your let-down will be negatively impacted.

Remember to always:

- Label your breast milk with the date and time you pumped it.
- Put your breast milk in the freezer and store by the date, using the oldest first.
- Once you take breast milk out of the freezer, remember you cannot refreeze it.
- To avoid problems, freeze your breast milk in smaller-size aliquots, no more than 4 ounces in 1 bag or bottle.

### Overactive Let-Down

In my breastfeeding practice, I see many mothers with overactive let-down. What is this and how do you know if you have it? These are my mamas who have an overactive and forceful milk ejection reflex. Many times, moms tell me that their milk shoots across the room or into the breast pump flange. Sometimes, the let-down can be painful. Because these babies are choking and gagging at the breast, they may be treated with reflux medications. Because of the increased foremilk these babies are getting, they can become gassy and have watery stools. Some babies may also clamp down on their mom's breast or try to pull off the breast as a way to manage and control the forceful let-down. Think of it as trying to drink from a garden hose; you'd be coughing and sputtering too!

Overactive let-down is a common source of frustration for both moms and babies. So what are the remedies to help fix this? Moms can hand express or use the electric pump to remove the initial let-down before offering the baby their breast. Also, changing positions can be helpful. I try to teach my moms to recline, in which you lay back slightly to remove the effect of gravity during the nursing session. As you become more comfortable, a side-lying pose is also helpful. Frequent burping throughout the feed will also help with your baby's symptoms.

I am here to tell you that nursing/breastfeeding/pumping is not easy during those early days and weeks. You may feel uncomfortable; your breasts may get very big; and they will feel, as I tell my moms, lumpy and bumpy. Often, depending on breast anatomy, feeding efficiency, and emptying of the breasts, you may feel areas that are more firm than other parts of the breast. This can lead to plugging of the ducts carrying your breast milk, which is normal to an extent. If this continues, it can lead to engorgement of that area of your breast. When you start feeling those harder areas, often located near your arm pits, start using your hands to massage those bumps out. You can do this while the baby is nursing, while you are on the pump, or even standing under the shower. While you're showering, do not soap up your nipples as this will cause them to become dry and even crack. If these steps don't work, take the back end of your electric toothbrush, turn it on, and allow that vibration to help break up the hardened area. If the situation doesn't improve, the bumps continue to get larger, there is redness in that area, and/or you develop a fever, you need to see your physician. Prolonged engorgement can lead to mastitis, which is a breast infection that requires antibiotic treatment.

## Importance of a Breast Self-Examination

When does a breast mass need to be evaluated?

While plugged ducts and engorgement are a normal part of breastfeeding, a breast lump or mass is not. Please do not ignore it. If you feel something during your breast self-examination, call your doctor to get it checked out right away.

## Formula Feeding

In some rare instances, medical conditions may prevent a baby from being able to receive breast milk. In this case, your baby will receive formula, and in some cases a specialized formula.

For my moms who are formula feeding, whether it is exclusively, partially, or when you are separated from your baby, I want to emphasize that you have nothing to feel bad or guilty about. Whether it's a personal decision for your physical or mental health or a medical necessity for your baby's health, it is OK. What I don't want you to get caught up in is the type of formula. Most of the formulas for healthy full-term infants are the same. I tell my mothers that it's like choosing between Coke and Pepsi. Please do not stress about the brand name or whether it is organic. Formula is expensive. I don't want you to feel as though you have to break the bank to afford a certain brand. If you are eligible for WIC, the Special Supplemental Nutrition Program for Women, Infants, and Children sponsored by the US Department of Agriculture, the formula company will be decided for you based on your state's contract. The only time we prescribe specialized formula is in cases of milk-protein allergy or sensitivities that the baby may have. These are specialized circumstances that your pediatrician will manage based on your baby's specific needs.

## How to Ask for Help

Whether you are nursing, pumping, or formula feeding, this is where you tell others how they can help you. Feeding a newborn is a full-time job. If you're nursing, have your partner bring the baby to you. Your partner/family member/doula can change the diaper before the feed or between sides to avoid waking the baby who may have fallen asleep while nursing. And of course, if the baby poops during the feed, please ask that person to burp the baby and change the diaper before placing the baby in the bassinet or crib to nap. If you're pumping, ask your family member to feed the baby expressed breast milk while you pump in another room. This is a great time for your partner to bond with the newborn and enjoy this uninterrupted time together. While my husband was feeding our daughter in another room, I pumped and read a magazine to catch up on the world around me! (This was before television streaming services.) Ask your partner to wash the pump parts or throw them in the dishwasher. If you are formula feeding, even if you are mixing the formula, show others how they can feed the baby while you rest or even take a shower. Remember, people can't read your mind, so please be vocal and tell those who are there to help you what you need.

## Food

Mamas often ask me about the foods they need to avoid if they are breastfeeding. Easy answer: none. When I was told after the birth of my first child that I had to avoid broccoli because it would cause her to be gassy, I was crushed. Chinese food from New York City was a staple of my diet. But no, vegetables won't make your baby gassy and you don't have to avoid spicy foods. I tell mamas that if they can tolerate it, so can the baby. In fact, for my mamas from other cultures, their ethnic foods, including the spices, are a great way for the baby to experience various flavors. Remember that your body needs an additional 450-500 calories per day as you breastfeed your baby. ACOG and the FDA recommend limiting fish and seafood consumption to 2-3 times a week, while avoiding fish with high mercury levels. This includes limiting albacore tuna to 6 ounces per week. If you eat fish caught in local water, checking for advisories about mercury is important, but if that information is not available, limit your fish/seafood intake to 1 serving or 6 ounces per week.

## Caffeine

Another important question I get is about caffeine intake. You do not have to completely stop your caffeine intake, whether it is from coffee, tea, or soda, while nursing. The recommended daily limit is 300 mg of caffeine, which translates to approximately 2 to 3 cups of coffee per day.

## *Alcohol*

What about drinking alcohol? Remember how I encouraged all of you to take time out for yourselves? That may be enjoying a cocktail with a girlfriend or a glass of wine with your partner for your first date night post-baby. I tell my mamas that 1 drink is safe while breastfeeding; the recommendation is to limit alcohol consumption to 2 drinks a week while nursing. Studies show that if you are going to have an alcoholic beverage, do so after you nurse your infant or immediately after pumping.

What is 1 drink? One drink is 12 ounces of beer, 5 ounces of wine, 1.5 ounces of distilled spirits/liquor. It generally takes 1 to 3 hours for the alcohol to be metabolized, so, if possible, wait 2 hours after you have had your glass of wine or a cocktail to nurse. A very small percentage of alcohol gets through the breast milk and will not hurt your baby. One thing I do *not* want you to do is "pump and dump." Pumping and dumping does *not* speed up the metabolism process in your body, so please do not

---

### Medications During Breastfeeding

This one still irks me. Every week, at least one mother tells me she was told by her physician, a pharmacist, or a family member that she will have to stop breastfeeding because the medication she has been taking or has been prescribed is unsafe while breastfeeding. Or moms are told to pump and dump for a certain amount of time before they can resume breastfeeding. If you are given a medication, please speak to a breastfeeding medicine specialist if you or the prescribing physician is unsure. Most medications are compatible with breastfeeding and will not cause any harm to your infant. There are free evidence-based resources such as LactMed (https://www.ncbi.nlm.nih.gov/books/NBK501922/) that all physicians, health care providers, and pharmacists can access when prescribing medication.

And, please, don't pump and dump; it makes me cry just thinking of all that liquid gold going down the drain.

do this. Enjoy your night out, relax, and you will see your baby when you get home.

## Unwanted Advice

Depending on various factors, whether societal, familial, racial, or cultural, you may receive unsolicited advice and pressure from others based on how and what you decide to feed your baby. I want to help you address this issue.

Remember when I shared that I couldn't nurse my first child? Well, I was at a religious ceremony feeding my baby a pumped bottle of milk. A woman who I did not even know, also with a young child, said to me, "I can't believe you are giving your baby a bottle." A female family member asked me, "Why are you doing so much work pumping? Just go ahead and give her formula."

Another family member commented, "If you don't nurse her, you will never be able to bond with her." I'll be honest, even writing this last one still fills me with sadness almost 20 years later.

When you make decisions about infant feeding, I want you to get advice that is evidence based. If you decide during pregnancy or even after delivery to breastfeed, that is fine. I want you to find the help and support you need to meet your breastfeeding goals. Just realize that those goals may change. Whether you want to go longer or stop sooner, either is fine. As I said earlier, some breastfeeding is better than none.

As every mother, baby, and situation are different, I often tell the mothers in my office this story, which will stop their tears as they begin to laugh.

> 66 It's OK, mama, if your baby gets some formula. It was so hard, my own baby was so small she needed formula. And guess what? She's 18, got into college, takes honors classes...but she still rolls her eyes. 99

What I do not want is for you to discontinue breastfeeding because you did not receive the support you needed in those early days. Or you stopped breastfeeding as a result of bad advice that had you question the safety of your feeding choice. *You* are in charge. I am here to give you information that will empower you, so you feel supported in the decisions that you make. I am here to remind you that only you know what will work for your baby and you. Ask for help. Relate your worries and concerns to your spouse, a family member, or a friend. You are not alone in these feelings, trust me. And remember, the way you choose to feed your baby is not a judgment about you, as a mother. Give yourself grace, mama!

# CHAPTER 8

# Postpartum Nutrition and Exercise

**EXERCISE**/noun/ˈeksərˌsīz/: activity requiring physical effort, carried out to sustain or improve health and fitness

Salads, yes salads. While I was nursing, pumping, doing laundry, and managing a newborn all by myself while my husband was at work, I was eating salads. Why? Not for the taste. Not because they gave me energy to get through my day. Nope. I was eating salads so I could start losing some of the 40 pounds I had gained during pregnancy and while on bed rest the last 2 months. I was on bed rest because my baby was too small and the maternal–fetal medicine specialist and obstetrician *wanted* me to gain weight. Gain weight so my baby would get bigger and stronger and not arrive too soon. But now she was home (thankfully!) and I felt frumpy, my boobs were huge, and, yes, I was still wearing my maternity stretch pants and bibs (maternity bibs were the "in thing" 19 years ago). My daughter was not even 1 month old. So what I had gained in about 6 months, I wanted to lose in 1.

I know many of you can relate to this story. I've seen this with my friends, colleagues, and so many mothers in my practice. That necessity to hurry up and lose the weight. The belief that we will return to our prepregnancy bodies almost immediately. Do we think that's the norm? Again, we are comparing ourselves to other mothers and thinking, *If she can do that, then why can't I?*

Although getting back to our healthy weight is important, the *way* we go about it is what is important. After all these years of being a mother, I still find the guidance on this issue severely lacking. New moms are trying to meet unrealistic expectations, which not only affects their physical health but also their mental health.

What's my mantra? Say it with me: *Happy and healthy mama equals happy and healthy baby.* This includes your immediate postpartum physical and mental health. It is *not* about being a certain size or a number on the scale. It is about maintaining your health after you just grew and gave birth to a human. Give yourself grace, mama.

## YOUR POSTPARTUM JOURNEY

Your postpartum journey, just like your pregnancy, will be unique to you. Whether it is how much weight you gained, how much your baby weighed, any health conditions or complications of pregnancy, your journey is your own. I know it is hard, but please stop comparing yourself to other moms, especially regarding your body shape.

Keep in mind, you were just pregnant (or if you received this book as a gift, you currently are pregnant). Your body was a haven for your baby growing inside of you. What you ate and drank, your physical movements, your emotions—*all* of it nurtured your baby, making him or her bigger and stronger until he or she was ready to come out into the world. Sounds pretty amazing, right? You're a superhero really. Mom-cape anyone?

Over the past 3 trimesters, you took care of yourself to maintain a healthy pregnancy so you would have a strong and healthy baby. Now, just because the baby is out of your body does not mean you get to neglect it in the fourth trimester.

> 66 I hate seeing the magazine covers at the grocery check-out aisle. I feel like they always have a picture of a celebrity mom who bounced back into her prebaby bod! Of course, I could do that if I had a nanny, a chef, and a maid. 99

## LET'S TALK ABOUT NUTRITION

Unfortunately, *dieting* is a commonly used word in our culture, and its use is not going to change anytime soon. But I would like you to reframe your thinking , which I know is difficult. Most *diets* fail. One statistic is that 95% of diets fail and most people regain their lost weight within 1 to 5 years. Sadly, 75% of American women surveyed admitted to having unhealthy thoughts, feelings, or behaviors related to food or their bodies. This is also true for postpartum women. If you're like most new moms, you're eager to put away your maternity clothes and slip into your old jeans. However, it's important to understand that approaching weight loss smartly and safely after pregnancy will not only help you with future pregnancies but will also promote good health throughout your life.

Healthy eating. Nutrition. Fueling your postpartum body. These are the terms I want you to keep in mind while reading this chapter. Fad diets (anyone heard of cayenne pepper and lemon water?), cutting out all carbs (even fruit!), supplements to quench your appetite. Many mamas have tried these quick fixes in the early postpartum period. I'll tell you right now that they don't work, not long-term anyway. Plus, they make you feel pretty lousy.

If you are reading this but also wondering how you can lose this baby weight, let me remind you, it is not about bouncing back immediately into your pre-baby body. And it's not about becoming a size zero. In this chapter, I give you a realistic way to become healthy and, if you desire, to lose the weight. We will strategize ways to eat healthfully while maintaining caloric intake for your physical health and your mental health as well as to strengthen your body. What you can't do is become hyperfocused about a number on a scale.

## Simple Steps for Healthy Eating

First, let's talk about some simple steps for healthy eating. During this early postpartum period, I discourage you from keeping track of calories and every spoonful you eat. I understand that, for some mamas, doing so is helpful. But, if it is burdensome, stresses you out, or causes you to become obsessive about a certain number, please put down your smartphone.

During your pregnancy, you were eating for 2, and understandably your eating habits changed to support your baby's growth. Not to mention those food cravings! Like I have said throughout this book (and will continue to say), just because the baby is now outside of your body, the 2 of you are still connected. Your nutrition and health are just as important while you care for your newborn, but they are also important to sustain and replenish your body after one of the most physically taxing experiences any human being can have—you grew, nourished, and birthed a baby. If you're breastfeeding, nutrition and hydration are essential to maintain your milk supply. Making healthy dietary choices will keep you in good health while allowing you to slowly lose your baby weight, if desired, and keep it off.

If you are breastfeeding, maintaining hydration and nutrition is essential, not just for you and your body but to maintain breast milk production. You will burn approximately 500 to 600 calories per day while breastfeeding, so you need to replace that energy. Eat healthy foods that are high in protein and remember to feed yourself while you are feeding your baby (refer to Chapter 7).

## Protein Intake

Intake of proteins is important, as these are the building blocks of your body. They help to repair your body and allow it to recover from the physiologic strain of pregnancy and childbirth. For my breastfeeding mamas, protein is important to help maintain your breast milk, which helps your baby's body and brain develop and grow. Whether you eat meat or are a vegetarian, it is recommended that approximately 25% of your daily calories come from protein. Again, do not pull out your calculators and apps. Try to eat 3 servings of protein daily. Whether it is plant based or animal based, lean protein is preferred over proteins that are fattier and higher in cholesterol. But do not deprive yourself, OK? If you want to have a juicy burger, go for it. Add some veggies on that patty and enjoy. Again, this is not meant to be restrictive, which is just a setup for failure, leading to increased frustration.

### Healthy Protein Options

Try to choose healthy proteins. Many of the foods in the following list can be packed and eaten on the go or when nursing. Make it easy on yourself and prepare accessible snacks in advance that you can grab at a moment's notice.

- Cheese
- Healthy nuts: almonds, walnuts, pistachios, cashews, and peanuts
- Seeds
- Protein bars
- Protein shakes
- Greek yogurt with granola
- Lean meats
- Eggs
- Fish

## *Fruits and Vegetables*

I know, I know, I know. Everyone talks about the importance of eating fruits and veggies. They are not only important for nutrition and revitalization of your body, but also a key component of healthy weight loss. I do not want you to worry about the carbohydrates in fruits. When the low-carb diet craze started years ago, fruit got a bad name. I saw friends and other women stop eating fruit completely because they had been told or had read that fruit was a source of carbohydrates.

## *Quick Nutrition Lesson*

I promise this won't be boring. Not all carbohydrates are created equal. The purpose of carbohydrates in our diet is to provide fuel for our bodies. When carbohydrates are broken down, they are transformed into glucose, which can be used as energy. They can also be turned into fat, which is stored for energy to be used later on.

You may have heard terms such as *complex* versus *simple carbohydrates* or *whole* versus refined. Let's break down the differences.

Simple or refined carbohydrates have been processed and the fiber has been removed or changed. Foods made with simple or refined carbohydrates include sugary beverages, sweets, white bread, and other foods made with white flour. Complex or whole carbohydrates are unprocessed and contain natural fiber. These foods include vegetables, fruits, legumes, and whole grains.

The big difference between these carbohydrates is that simple or refined carbs tend to cause a spike in blood sugar levels and, in turn, an insulin spike (which can subsequently store fat). However, what goes up must come down. After that initial feel-good sugar spike, there will be a crash in your blood sugar level that will cause you to feel hungry and unsatisfied and will lead you to crave more food. Maybe even more sugary snacks. Most of us can attest to that initial feel-good endorphin rush of a cookie or candy bar, but then feel hungry again within an hour.

In addition, these carbs do not contain essential nutrients; they are basically empty calories.

I am not telling you to stop eating refined carbs, but eating more whole carbs—making them a part of your nutrition throughout the day—will help you feel fuller longer, will keep you feeling satisfied, and is good for your overall health and metabolism. The key is moderation. So, no, I am not saying that you cannot have ice cream once in a while. What kind of friend would that make me? I'm a vanilla ice cream with extra hot fudge gal. But I digress.

In the immediate postpartum period, I do *not* want you to feel like you have to limit how much you eat. Your body is going to be tired, and you are going to be sleep-deprived. And hungry, which is normal. Instead of reaching for a candy bar, maybe grab a piece of fruit or vegetable that you can hold in one hand while juggling the baby with the other. Remember, it has to be easy to access throughout the day, especially for my mamas who may be home alone with a newborn.

### Meal Planning

Many of you may not like this, but planning will be super helpful. I realize that the term *meal planning* may feel daunting and cause you stress, but don't think of it as an elaborate task. Whether it's the night before or after that early morning feed while the baby is napping, plan out what you will eat over the next few hours. Make snack-size bags with healthy options that you can grab when hunger strikes. For those of you who have a partner living with you, family members staying with you, or friends stopping by, you need to recruit them for this specific task. Because your partner cannot read your mind or your friend may not know you're hungry while home alone all day, you must tell them your needs. Yes, they are holding the baby so you can take a shower or feeding the baby so you can take a quick nap. Feeding you is something your friends and family will not only enjoy doing but, as a bonus, it will take a major burden off your plate.

Let your partner, family members, and friends know what you need. Whether it's telling them your dietary restrictions and allergies, asking your partner to prepare a healthy meal for you after work, or asking your friend to pick up your favorite ingredients so you can make a protein shake that will be easy to sip while you're nursing, please do not hesitate to express your needs. What you are putting into your body is just as important during this fourth trimester as it was during the first 3 trimesters.

While this may seem obvious, you are probably not drinking enough water. Whether or not you are trying to lose weight, hydration is important as your body heals. For my breastfeeding mamas, hydration is important for the breast milk supply. Forget those small plastic water bottles that become warm sitting next to you all day (not to mention they're terrible for the environment). If you don't already have one, consider buying one of those large stainless-steel water bottles. Fill it with ice and water. It won't spill and you can carry it around in your free hand. Remember to drink between 50 and 60 ounces of water every day. Yes, you read that correctly and, no, you won't float away, I promise. This will keep you hydrated. Also, many times feelings of hunger are actually thirst, so drinking water before and after eating your snack or meal may actually help reduce unnecessary and unhealthy snacking.

## EXERCISE

While nutrition is a key component of your postpartum recovery, so is exercise. However, this does not mean you have to go back to your gym or that you need to run a few miles every day. It just means you have to get your body slowly moving again, which is good not only for your physical health but also for your mental health and well-being.

Do not jump back into your old exercise regimen. Doing so may not only cause injury or increased postpartum pain, but excessive and rapid physical activity can lead to increased postpartum bleeding or other complications after a vaginal or cesarean delivery.

First and foremost, any type of physical activity must be cleared by your obstetrician. Period. Depending on your level of activity during the pregnancy plus any complications during the pregnancy or after delivery, your physician will give you the green light. Resuming physical activity is different for everyone. It will vary among individuals based on certain factors, but it will even change for the same woman between children. Again, each pregnancy and each postpartum period, just like your child(ren), is different. Remember, this is not a race.

Not only has your life changed with this precious baby, but your body has too. Acknowledge that, recognize that, and appreciate that. To this day, 3 kids later, I look at my cesarean delivery scar as my battle scar. It reminds me of how strong I am. How I gave birth to 3 kids. My scar is a reminder of how amazingly strong my body is.

### Listening to Your Body

Initially, just getting out of bed may be painful for many of you. I see this with my mamas in my practice. My heart breaks for them as they struggle to walk into the office for the baby's initial checkup, with swollen feet and pain after delivery. Listen to your body. Control the pain with whatever your physician has given you. Do not be a martyr. Do not wait for the pain to become excruciating before you take your medication. However, make sure the medication is safe for breastfeeding, and if you are unsure, ask your physician. You do not have to choose between controlling your pain and breastfeeding.

The reason I am telling you this is because I made this exact mistake after my second baby. We moved while I was pregnant, so, of course, after delivery with a toddler running around and my husband back at work, I had to use my "free time" to unpack, right? If that meant lifting some small boxes, so be it. Guess what? Not only did I feel lousy, but I started bleeding and pretty heavily. Needless to say, my obstetrician was not too happy with me. But I learned my lesson and the boxes waited. All I am trying to say is that you need to listen to your body and not overdo it. Remember, your body needs to heal.

When your obstetrician gives you the green light to resume physical activity, start slowly. This goes for my marathon runners too. Be realistic. Incorporating physical activity into your daily routine helps you both physically and mentally. Start with a short walk with your baby. Whether it's pushing the baby in a stroller or carrying the baby in a wrap, getting outside in the fresh air will feel amazing, not to mention it will lull your baby to sleep. Eventually, you can work up to longer walks or even a faster pace. Start with small simple exercises that will help you strengthen major muscle groups. This does not mean you will do 100 sit-ups that first day, but slowly strengthening your abdominal and back muscles is important for your core strength, which will aid in your recovery. Gradually work up from there in time and intensity.

If you are rested, there are many short exercise routines available online that can be done in the house while your baby sleeps. Or for some of you, when someone comes over or your partner gets home, this is a great opportunity for you to head out for a short run or get on a bike at the gym. I encourage you to include your baby, whether it's going for a walk or placing the baby in a swing while you work out at home. Please don't feel that you are limited, especially if you don't have someone to care for the baby. You don't have to do it alone either. Whether it's a local mommy stroller group or a postpartum exercise class, for many women, having others around is motivating. Don't forget that water bottle, and remember to drink enough water before, during, and after your workout. If you experience any pain while exercising, please listen to your body and stop and rest. You don't want to overdo it.

For my breastfeeding mamas, nurse your baby or pump your breasts to avoid pain and discomfort from breast engorgement. Invest in a supportive bra that is correctly sized for your post-partum breasts, which will most likely be larger. After your workout, remove your sports bra as the tightness may cause some ductal blockage, leading to engorgement.

Returning to your prepregnancy body is important. I under-stand that. I really do. But please be realistic about your goals. Regarding weight loss, it is reasonable to lose anywhere between 0.5 and 1 pound a week. In terms of exercise, you will return to the level and intensity of activity you had before, but it will take some time, which is OK. Your body just did something incredible. The human body is amazing, so take care of it.

**CHAPTER 9**

# Postpartum Depression and Anxiety

*Trigger Warning: This chapter will discuss depression, anxiety, and other mood disorders. If you think you may be experiencing any of these conditions, please speak to your physician or call 911.*

**DEPRESSION**/dəˈpreSH(ə)n/noun: health condition characterized by feelings of severe despondency and dejection, typically also with feelings of inadequacy and guilt, often accompanied by lack of energy and disturbance of appetite and sleep

**ANXIETY**/aNGˈzīədē/noun: a feeling of worry, nervousness, or unease, typically about an imminent event or something with an uncertain outcome

**MOOD**/mo͞od/noun: a temporary state of mind or feeling

After moving to Virginia shortly after my third child was born, I was back at work and helping to plan a conference about postpartum depression and anxiety for doctors, nurses, and other health care professionals who work with new mothers and babies. Right before the lunch break, a panel of mothers were asked to share their own personal stories about their pregnancy and postpartum journeys. We explained to the audience that we were not allowing a question and answer session at the end. The guest speakers were telling their own stories, without interruption, which gave them a safe space to share. I sat in the front row, keeping an eye on the clock because, as the moderator, I needed to make sure everything stayed on schedule and nobody raised their hand to ask a question. Listening intently, I began to tear up, right there in the front row. It hit me right then and there, listening to these moms talk. What I had experienced 4 years earlier, after the birth of my second child, was not a feeling of being overwhelmed or just really tired because I had 2 kids in diapers. I realized, in that moment, that all those years ago, I had experienced postpartum depression. However, unlike these mothers, neither my husband nor I knew how to get the help I needed.

As a physician, I see lots of patients every day. A patient with a preterm baby came to see me for that first newborn visit. Because of that mom and baby, I started to realize that mom's postpartum mental health (actually, her mental health even *during* the pregnancy) does not receive enough attention, and this aspect of the fourth trimester is often missed. The more I read and learned, the more intense my interest became. I realized that mom's mental health and well-being are *directly* linked not only to her overall health but also to that of her baby. This is a time of intense emotion and dramatic change in a woman's life. We need to acknowledge this and provide greater support for all mothers.

Honestly, the fact that mom's and baby's mental and physical health are so connected is not rocket science. You carried that child for 9 months; is it surprising that the baby depends on you after your delivery? In those early days, weeks, and months, *you* are the primary caregiver for that newborn. This is not to say that your spouse/partner, family member, babysitter, or friend is not a big part of your baby's care, but mom is the number 1 person for that baby. While that mother-child connection can feel precious and priceless at times, being the primary person responsible for your new baby can also sometimes feel like overwhelming pressure. At times, mothers are not sure if they even feel that bond and worry that they are not cut out to be good mothers as a result. These feelings and concerns are common, especially among those mothers experiencing postpartum anxiety and depression. But whether you have some risk factors or none, postpartum depression and anxiety, also known as postpartum mood and anxiety disorders, is *the* most common complication of childbirth and affects up to 25% of mothers. And it can significantly affect the health and well-being of mothers, their infants, and families.

## THE POSTPARTUM SPECTRUM OF PSYCHIATRIC SYNDROMES

### *Postpartum Blues*

The postpartum spectrum of psychiatric syndromes can be classified into 3 major categories: postpartum blues, postpartum psychosis, and postpartum depression. *Postpartum blues* are a common emotional experience for women after delivery, affecting up to 80% of women. Symptoms of postpartum blues include emotional imbalance, difficulty sleeping, decreased appetite, and excessive anxiety. These feelings typically begin within the first 5 days after delivery and sometimes resolve on their own by day 14.

### *Postpartum Psychosis*

*Postpartum psychosis* is a psychiatric emergency that occurs in the first month. It must be addressed immediately and mom needs to be taken to the hospital. Symptoms include substantial mood shifts, paranoia, hallucinations, delusions, and suicidal or homicidal thoughts, which may put mom and/or the newborn at risk. Although the incidence of psychosis is extremely low, women with a history of bipolar disorder have a higher risk of developing postpartum psychosis. However, some women who develop postpartum psychosis have no previous psychiatric history. Postpartum psychosis is a psychiatric emergency, and those around mom (partner/family member/friend) must promptly get her to the closest emergency department.

## Postpartum Depression

*Postpartum depression* occurs at delivery or within the first 4 months after delivery and can last several months to a year and can range from mild to severe. Although postpartum mood and anxiety disorders are common, the variation in timing and symptoms, along with other conditions, such as anxiety and bipolar disorder, can complicate the diagnosis.

Many new mothers experience trouble sleeping, weight loss, exhaustion, anxiety, loss of interest in usual activities, and depressed mood. However, with postpartum depression, the symptoms last longer and generally are more severe than those in moms with postpartum blues. Postpartum depression and anxiety last longer than 2 weeks, symptoms can occur daily, and they can cause functional impairment with daily activities, including caring for your newborn and yourself.

Postpartum depression and anxiety can range from mild to severe. However, based on certain risk factors, some mothers will be more likely to develop postpartum depression and/or postpartum anxiety. Untreated anxiety and/or depression during pregnancy puts moms at a greater risk of developing postpartum anxiety and/or depression. Other factors that increase the likelihood of developing postpartum depression and/or anxiety are young maternal age, lower socioeconomic status, lack of social support, unplanned pregnancy, psychosocial stress from partner/spouse, alcohol or substance abuse, and a family history of depression. However, even if you have none of these risk factors, you can still develop a postpartum mood disorder. Remember, it is the most common complication of childbirth. But with proper support, guidance, and resources, you will get better, leading to improved outcomes for both you and your baby.

# INTRUSIVE THOUGHTS

A distinct aspect of postpartum mood disorders that we do not find with major depressive disorder or generalized anxiety disorder outside of the perinatal or postpartum period is something called *intrusive thoughts*. I think everyone who works with pregnant moms, new moms, and newborns during the postpartum period should be aware of these symptoms, not only because they are common, but also because they can be downright scary. Intrusive or obsessive thoughts are involuntary thoughts or subconscious ideas that can become repetitive and compulsive in nature. These stressful thoughts can be difficult to control and eliminate for new moms. We often refer to them as *ego-dystonic,* meaning that these are part of your subconscious and do not reflect your actual thoughts; basically, these are thoughts that pop into your head, and as a new mom, you do not want them there. An example of an intrusive thought is a mother envisioning hurting her infant. Other examples I've heard are the following: "What if I accidentally fall down the stairs while holding my baby?" "What if I accidentally let go of my baby while bathing her?" "What if I accidentally drive off the road?" These thoughts are common; in fact, some studies show that 85% of women experience them in the postpartum period. The fear is not only that these things could happen, but that somehow you may subconsciously do something like that on purpose.

A close friend uttered these words to me when I was talking about my work with postpartum mothers. She said that during the entire time she was experiencing these thoughts, she told no one. Not her doctor, her baby's pediatrician, her mother, her best friend, or

> 66
>
> I was so scared, I couldn't even tell my husband.
> I thought I was going crazy.
> 99

her husband. The thought of my mamas feeling this fear and terror while believing that something is wrong with them and then being too scared to ask for help just breaks my heart.

If any of you reading this have ever experienced intrusive thoughts, I am so sorry. If anyone reading this is currently experiencing them, please reach out for help (see Resources for Moms). These thoughts are a normal part of postpartum depression/anxiety and are not a sign that you are experiencing postpartum psychosis or that you are an unfit mother. I don't want any of my mothers to think that their baby will be taken away from them. What is most important is for you to get the help you need.

### Screening

The American College of Obstetricians and Gynecologists recommends that a mother should be screened at least once during pregnancy and at their 6-week postpartum checkup with their obstetrician. Can I rant a little? If moms can start experiencing postpartum depression and/or anxiety within the first week or 2 after delivery, how is seeing your obstetrician and getting screened for postpartum depression/postpartum anxiety sufficient at the 6-week mark? Do not get me wrong; this is *not* the fault of your obstetrician. As I've mentioned time and time again, in the United States at least, visits and payments for these visits are controlled by the health insurance companies. Many of us across the fields of obstetrics and pediatrics continue to fight on a legislative and policy level for moms to receive more frequent and individualized postpartum care.

You're probably thinking that if depression and anxiety are so common and I don't see my physician until 6 weeks after delivery, who is going to help me if I need it before then? First, let me start by saying that you do not need a professional to screen you to be diagnosed and get help. The resources listed at the end of this chapter include sites you can access to get the help you need without waiting.

To address this issue, the American Academy of Pediatrics recommends that all pediatricians/pediatric health care providers first screen by the baby's 1-month well-child check, followed by screening at the 2-month, 4-month, and 6-month checkups. However, please note that not all pediatricians feel comfortable screening or have all the information needed to screen mothers for postpartum depression/anxiety. Still, if your pediatrician doesn't automatically screen, please ask. Feel free to show the pediatrician this page and talk about all of your questions and concerns. The more that physicians know, the better. When other physicians in my health care system started screening, they were shocked to find out how many of their mothers were experiencing it and *never* knew. They were grateful to be made aware so they could help their mamas and babies.

When I started screening, based on what I was seeing in my practice, I actually wanted to begin earlier, and we now screen at the 2-week weight-check visit. As a result, we find more mothers who are at risk, and the clinical protocol is now being used across our entire health system as well as in our neonatal intensive care unit for moms of our preterm babies.

When pediatricians screen for postpartum depression/anxiety, most use the Edinburgh Postnatal Depression Scale (EPDS). What is important to know is that while the tool does not diagnose postpartum depression/anxiety, it helps us determine if you are at risk. The scale also allows us to follow your progress and improvement once you receive help. Using the EPDS table on pages 100 and 101, you also can screen yourself and then ask for the help you need. As you can see, the questions on the EPDS ask about a variety of symptoms, and the final question asks about any harmful thoughts. Since starting to screen in my practice 11 years ago, I have observed that moms are predominantly honest, even with that last question because they *want* to talk about it, they want help. They want to be heard. And even

# Edinburgh Postnatal Depression Scale

You can screen yourself using the Edinburgh Postnatal Depression Scale below. (It's freely available at https://www.fresno.ucsf.edu/pediatrics/downloads/edinburghscale.pdf.)

## Edinburgh Postnatal Depression Scale[1] (EPDS)

Name:_____     Address: _____

Your Date of Birth: _____     _____

Baby's Date of Birth:_____     Phone:  _____

As you are pregnant or have recently had a baby, we would like to know how you are feeling. Please check the answer that comes closest to how you have felt IN THE PAST 7 DAYS, not just how you feel today.

Here is an example, already completed.

I have felt happy:
- ☐ Yes, all the time
- ☒ Yes, most of the time     This would mean: "I have felt happy most of the time" during the past week.
- ☐ No, not very often     Please complete the other questions in the same way.
- ☐ No, not at all

In the past 7 days:

1. I have been able to laugh and see the funny side of things
   - ☐ As much as I always could
   - ☐ Not quite so much now
   - ☐ Definitely not so much now
   - ☐ Not at all

2. I have looked forward with enjoyment to things
   - ☐ As much as I ever did
   - ☐ Rather less than I used to
   - ☐ Definitely less than I used to
   - ☐ Hardly at all

*3. I have blamed myself unnecessarily when things went wrong
   - ☐ Yes, most of the time
   - ☐ Yes, some of the time
   - ☐ Not very often
   - ☐ No, never

4. I have been anxious or worried for no good reason
   - ☐ No, not at all
   - ☐ Hardly ever
   - ☐ Yes, sometimes
   - ☐ Yes, very often

*5. I have felt scared or panicky for no very good reason
   - ☐ Yes, quite a lot
   - ☐ Yes, sometimes
   - ☐ No, not much
   - ☐ No, not at all

*6. Things have been getting on top of me
   - ☐ Yes, most of the time I haven't been able to cope at all
   - ☐ Yes, sometimes I haven't been coping as well as usual
   - ☐ No, most of the time I have coped quite well
   - ☐ No, I have been coping as well as ever

*7. I have been so unhappy that I have had difficulty sleeping
   - ☐ Yes, most of the time
   - ☐ Yes, sometimes
   - ☐ Not very often
   - ☐ No, not at all

*8. I have felt sad or miserable
   - ☐ Yes, most of the time
   - ☐ Yes, quite often
   - ☐ Not very often
   - ☐ No, not at all

*9. I have been so unhappy that I have been crying
   - ☐ Yes, most of the time
   - ☐ Yes, quite often
   - ☐ Only occasionally
   - ☐ No, never

*10. The thought of harming myself has occurred to me
   - ☐ Yes, quite often
   - ☐ Sometimes
   - ☐ Hardly ever
   - ☐ Never

Administered/Reviewed by_____Date _____

[1] Source: Cox, JL., Holden, JM., and Sagovsky, R. 1987. Detection of postnatal depression: Development of the 10-item Edinburgh Postnatal Depression Scale.     British Journal of Psychiatry 150:782-786 .

[2] Source: K. L. Wisner, B. L. Parry, C. M. Piontek, Postpartum Depression N Engl JMed vol. 347, No 3, July 18, 2002, 194-199

Users may reproduce the scale without further permission providing they respect copyright by quoting the names of the authors, the title and the source of the paper in all reproduced copies.

## Edinburgh Postnatal Depression Scale[1] (EPDS)

Postpartum depression is the most common complication of childbearing.[2] The 10-question Edinburgh Postnatal Depression Scale (EPDS) is a valuable and efficient way of identifying patients at risk for "perinatal" depression. The EPDS is easy to administer and has proven to be an effective screening tool.

Mothers who score above 13 are likely to be suffering from a depressive illness of varying severity. The EPDS score should not override clinical judgment. A careful clinical assessment should be carried out to confirm the diagnosis. The scale indicates how the mother has felt during the previous week. In doubtful cases it may be useful to repeat the tool after 2 weeks. The scale will not detect mothers with anxiety neuroses, phobias or personality disorders.

## Scoring

### QUESTIONS 1, 2, & 4 (without an *)

Are scored 0, 1, 2 or 3 with top box scored as 0 and the bottom box scored as 3.

### QUESTIONS 3, 5-10 (marked with an *)

Are reverse scored, with the top box scored as a 3 and the bottom box scored as 0.

Maximum score: 30

Possible Depression: 10 or greater
Always look at item 10 (suicidal thoughts)

**Instructions for using the Edinburgh Postnatal Depression Scale:**

1. The mother is asked to check the response that comes closest to how she has been feeling in the previous 7 days.

2. All the items must be completed.

3. Care should be taken to avoid the possibility of the mother discussing her answers with others. (Answers come from the mother or pregnant woman.)

4. The mother should complete the scale herself, unless she has limited English or has difficulty with reading.

though the scale cannot diagnose postpartum depression in any of my mamas, it helps me start the conversation with zero judgment. My hope is that universal screening during well-child (health supervision) visits will help reduce the stigma associated with postpartum depression/anxiety, regardless of whether you are a new mom or a seasoned mom with 3 children. On a personal and professional level, I know that postpartum depression/anxiety can affect *any one* of us as mothers. You are not alone and there is absolutely nothing to be ashamed of. You are not a bad mother. You are a strong and nurturing mama taking care of yourself and your new baby. Please don't ever forget that!

Postpartum depression is increasingly becoming recognized as more high-profile women, such as Brooke Shields, Serena Williams, and Bryce Howard, are talking about their experiences; however, postpartum mood disorders do not always present as sadness or a tearful mother. More often than not, they present with symptoms of anxiety or severe worry.

Moms with postpartum anxiety and excessive worry typically say things like this:

> 66 My daughter got sick and I had to take her to the emergency room 3 times last week, and the doctors said there is nothing wrong with her. I don't get it, when she's with my husband, she is OK. 99

Moms with feelings of anxiety about the baby's safety are unable to sleep or rest while the baby sleeps:

> 66 Even when she sleeps, I can't rest. I check to make sure she's breathing or I scroll through Facebook and see these moms who are doing everything right. 99

## Getting Help

I have heard these statements and others from many moms, both in my practice as well as from friends and acquaintances who confide in me when they find out I am a pediatrician. Postpartum anxiety is extremely common; in fact, postpartum anxiety is often more prevalent than postpartum depression and is the most common postpartum mood disorder that many mothers face. Often, anxiety and depression occur at the same time. Excessive worry, inability to rest, continued worrying that can be debilitating are all signs that a mom may be experiencing postpartum anxiety. Please do not ignore these symptoms just because you are not feeling sad, hopeless, or tearful. Every mom and every postpartum period is different. Please understand that you are not alone and that it is OK to ask for help.

This was me. Asking for help from my obstetrician, who also was a friend. Instead of listening to me and my concerns, the obstetrician shut me out. To say I was devastated is an understatement. I

> ❝ I called my obstetrician's office because I wasn't feeling right. I didn't know what to do, and my husband didn't either. When I told the nurse that I was feeling so sad and hopeless, she put me on hold to chat with the doctor. She came back and told me to call the number on the back of my insurance card to get help. And then she hung up. ❞

felt sad. I felt angry. I felt ashamed. And you know what? Because of that conversation (back in 2004), I was so dejected that I never asked for help again. It was only years later, as I sat in the front row of our conference, that I realized what I had been going through. So, when I saw mamas in my practice having the same experience, I decided to help ensure that other mothers wouldn't go through what I (and so many others) had before. Because of societal, familial, and cultural expectations, mamas, especially in that fourth trimester, are supposed to do it all, never ask for help, and stuff our emotions as we care for and feed a newborn while juggling everything else in our lives. I am here to tell you that that is a fictitious standard that is not sustainable.

So where can you start? First and foremost, you need to reach out to someone you can trust—a partner, family member, friend, or neighbor—and explain how you're feeling and that you need help. Believe me, I know how difficult it is to ask for help. But whether it's asking a friend to watch the baby so you can get some sleep, attending a support group, or asking your doctor for help, remember to celebrate the fact that you are taking steps to care for yourself and your baby.

After you talk with someone you trust, call your obstetrician or the health care professional who delivered your baby. Perhaps after being examined, your doctor will suggest therapy as the first step. Depending on your medical history and your needs, he or she can refer you for therapy and may even prescribe medications you previously were on, if necessary. If you have a history of mood disorders, please contact your therapist and psychiatrist if you had been seeing one.

Peer support is another important piece of the puzzle. As a result of the COVID-19 global pandemic, accessing support groups has become easier because many of these resources are now virtual. You don't have to talk and you don't have to share if you're not ready. But believe me, meeting (even virtually) and listening to other mamas just like you will help you feel less alone. There is no judgment, as every woman in the support group has experienced or is currently experiencing much of what you are feeling.

One important point I'd like to stress for my pregnant mamas. If you have anxiety and/or depression during this pregnancy or have a history of anxiety and/or depression, do *not* stop your medications. Please talk with your obstetrician about any concerns you may have about taking medications while you are pregnant. Untreated depression or anxiety during pregnancy is *the* most significant risk factor for developing these same symptoms in the postpartum period. I see this time and time again in my practice. Whether your concerns are based on a recommendation from a physician, therapist, family member, or friend, or perhaps this is how you are feeling about this issue, please do not stop your medication without speaking to your obstetrician.

Unfortunately, I see pregnant mothers who either stop taking their psychiatric medications or decrease the dosage because of fear of harming their unborn babies. Even though there is little scientific evidence linking these medications to any harmful effects on the fetus, pregnant women are terrified of harm coming to their unborn child. Physicians and other health care providers who work with pregnant women need to know the evidence and discuss the risks and benefits of medication with their patients. If your physician is not comfortable managing your psychiatric medications during and/or after your pregnancy, ask for the name of a perinatal psychiatrist. But no one, whether a physician, family member, or friend, should tell a woman to completely stop taking her psychiatric medication and just hang on and wait for these feelings to pass.

I ask my moms this question: If you had asthma or high blood pressure or diabetes, would you suddenly stop taking your medications and "just get through" that asthma attack, that bout of high blood pressure, or those high insulin readings? Of course not! So, if you wouldn't stop medications for your physical health during pregnancy, why would you do that for your mental health? Last time I checked, the brain and body were connected. Again, please speak with your obstetrician or ask for a referral to a perinatal psychiatrist to help manage your treatment during your pregnancy and even after the baby is born during the postpartum period.

Once you've reached out to a friend, logged into a virtual support group for postpartum depression/anxiety, and are waiting for your doctor to call you back, what else can you do? This may sound ridiculous for me to say to a mom with a newborn, but you need to sleep. Getting 5 to 6 hours of uninterrupted sleep can and will drastically improve your mood, regardless of the severity of your symptoms. Now you're thinking, how does she expect me to get 5 hours of sleep with a newborn? Although I will go into depth in Chapter 15, this is where you will (again) enlist the help of a parent, friend, family member, neighbor, or someone else you trust in your home with your newborn. Or maybe some of you have the means to hire help, such as a postpartum doula, night nurse, nanny, or babysitter. Although you need to sleep and rest when the baby rests, that 5- to 6-hour stretch of uninterrupted sleep is really important. Consider nursing or feeding your baby, after which you go to your bed and sleep alone. While you sleep, someone else burps and changes your baby. The next bottle feed for your baby should be handed over to the person who is in your home to help. This goes for my breastfeeding mamas too. Whether it's a bottle of pumped breast milk or a bottle of formula, let someone you trust feed your newborn so you can get uninterrupted sleep. For my formula-feeding mamas, this can occur for another feed as well. My breastfeeding mothers will wake up for that next feed to nurse or pump, thereby preventing engorgement and breast pain.

I always tell my moms and their partners that once mom feeds or nurses the newborn, step in and take the baby (and any older sibling) out of the house for a short time. Go for a walk so your older child can get some much-needed exercise. Often, it is very difficult for moms to sleep soundly when the baby is nearby. Mamas, don't feel guilty asking your partner, family member, or friend to take the baby out—believe me, the baby will sleep well with a full belly while being pushed in a stroller. Remember to communicate what you need.

## BREASTFEEDING AND POSTPARTUM DEPRESSION/ANXIETY: TO TREAT OR NOT TO TREAT

Many moms feel that they have to choose between breastfeeding and receiving treatment for their postpartum depression/anxiety. Not only do my mamas feel guilty, but, sadly, there is still a lot of misinformation out there. Not to mention the fear-inducing commercials and news articles that discuss use of psychiatric medication during pregnancy and while breastfeeding. Again, another reason for this book: evidence-based medicine, not internet opinion or fear-mongering misinformation. Many fear that taking medication while breastfeeding could harm their babies, while others fear the stigma associated with a diagnosis of postpartum depression/anxiety. Some women believe that accepting a diagnosis will mean they are bad moms and that perinatal mood disorders are something you just need to get through while you're breastfeeding.

Although some moms are still being told to choose between breastfeeding and treatment, thankfully, things are changing. Obstetricians and psychiatrists are becoming more comfortable treating breastfeeding mothers who have postpartum

> 66 I work in health care and I knew that something wasn't right. But I didn't want to tell my doctor or see a therapist because I knew they'd tell me I'd have to start medication and stop breastfeeding. And that is something I could not do. My birth didn't go the way I wanted, so for me, I had to breastfeed, and my goal was to get to 1 year. 99

depression/anxiety. This is great news because, with various initiatives and screening protocols, more and more mothers who are experiencing postpartum depression will be identified earlier and receive the help they need.

I counsel mothers that the medications usually used to treat postpartum depression and anxiety are safe to take while breastfeeding. This class of drugs, known as selective serotonin reuptake inhibitors (SSRIs), has been around a long time, giving us a great deal of information about its safety profile. In fact, some colleagues and I published an article entitled "Use of Antidepressants in Breastfeeding Mothers, ABM Clinical Protocol #18" to help educate physicians and health care professionals so they have access to the evidence when treating postpartum mental health conditions in breastfeeding mothers (access freely at https://www.bfmed.org/assets/DOCUMENTS/PROTOCOLS/ 18-use-of-antidepressants-protocol-english.pdf).

No one should tell a mother who has postpartum depression or anxiety that she has to choose between medication and breastfeeding. This is not only irresponsible and incorrect, but also dangerous. Please find a knowledgeable physician so you can get the help you need while achieving your breastfeeding goals.

What about my mamas for whom breastfeeding is exacerbating their postpartum depression/anxiety? While evidence
shows that breastfeeding can be protective, as a pediatrician, I
am also in the position of supporting moms who decide to *stop*
breastfeeding. What if breastfeeding is worsening her ability to
sleep, increasing her anxiety, and generally making her mental
health worse? There is no shame in feeding your baby formula.
For many moms, receiving this validation that they can stop
breastfeeding is a relief and, hopefully, minimizes their guilt. As
a pediatrician, I care for babies, but my goal is also to empower
mothers to do what is best for their babies, while taking care
of themselves. What's my mantra? Say it with me: *A happy and
healthy mama equals a happy and healthy baby.*

| Resources for Moms | |
| --- | --- |
| **Organizations** | **Websites** |
| **National Suicide Pre-vention Lifeline** <br> 1-800-273-8255 | www.suicidepreventionlifeline.org |
| **Postpartum Support International** <br> 1-800-944-4773 | https://www.postpartum.net/ |
| **American Academy of Pediatrics** | www.healthychildren.org/English/ ages-stages/prenatal/Pages/ Depression-and-Anxiety-During-Preg-nancy-and-After-Birth-FAQs.aspx |

| | |
|---|---|
| **American College of Obstetricians and Gynecologists** | https://www.acog.org/womens-health/faqs/postpartum-depression |
| **Academy of Breast-feeding Medicine** | www.bfmed.org/find-a-physician#/ |
| **Medications for Depression and Anxiety While Breastfeeding** | www.bfmed.org/assets/DOCUMENTS/PROTOCOLS/18-use-of-antidepressants-protocol-english.pdf |
| **MotherToBaby** | https://mothertobaby.org/pregnancy-breastfeeding-exposures/anxiety/ |
| **SAMHSA: Substance Abuse and Mental Health Services Administration** 1-800-662-HELP (4357) | www.samhsa.gov/find-help/national-helpline |
| **National Alliance on Mental Illness** 1-800-950-6264 In a crisis, text NAME to 741741 | www.nami.org/Home |
| **Centers for Disease Control and Prevention** | www.cdc.gov/reproductivehealth/depression/resources.htm |

## Postpartum Rage

Postpartum rage is real and although less common than post-partum depression/anxiety can affect many moms. Symptoms to look for include:

- Difficulty controlling your temper
- Screaming, swearing, punching, throwing things
- Violent thoughts directed toward your partner/spouse or other family members
- Dwelling on situations that continue to upset you, unable to "snap out of it"

Postpartum rage is often unrecognized and not discussed, but this does not mean these feelings aren't real. For my mamas experiencing symptoms of postpartum rage, you need to reach out and ask for help, including from a family member or a friend. More importantly, reach out to your physician, talk to a therapist, and, if needed, start taking medication. Do not feel shame or that you have done something wrong. With help and guidance, you will feel better.

## Why Do I Feel Sad and Worried During my Let-down?

Dysphoric Milk Ejection Reflex, also known as D-MER, occurs right before milk release and only lasts a few minutes. Moms may experience feelings of sadness, anxiety, and even self-loathing. There is a physiologic reason for this. These feelings are caused by the various hormones released during breastfeeding and are completely normal. While they can be frustrating to you during this special bonding time with your new baby, please know you are doing nothing wrong.

One important point to keep in mind is that D-MER is transient and should last only a few minutes. If you have persistent feelings of sadness or anxiety, please speak to someone and receive the proper evaluation and treatment you need from your doctor.

## A Special Note for my Latina Mothers:
## Mal de Nervios

For many Latina mothers, symptoms of depression/anxiety in the postpartum period are often attributed to bad nerves rather than being recognized as a physiologic condition of pregnancy and motherhood. Because of some cultural and familial beliefs, there is a strong expectation to be a good mother and always put the baby first, even if this means ignoring mom's health. For many communities, feeling overwhelmed, sad, and worried are part of being a mother and the woman just needs to get through it.

This information is important for those who work with Latina mothers because they may manifest their symptoms of depression/anxiety differently from other patients and may be less willing to accept help, whether it is through support groups, therapy, or medication, because doing so may not be culturally acceptable. Again, it is important to discuss postpartum depression/anxiety with all mothers to raise awareness while reducing any stigma for those moms who may be reluctant to ask for help.

> **❝** Remember, mothers, you are not alone, you are not to blame, and with help you will get well **❞**

CHAPTER 10

# Return to You

> **RETURN**/verb/rəˈtərn: come or go back to a place or person
> noun/ an act of coming or going back to a place or activity

We've talked about postpartum breasts and postpartum brains, and now I want to talk about your postpartum body. The human body is amazing. Well, let me add that the *female* body is amazing. Before pregnancy, the uterus is about the size and shape of an upside-down pear. By the ninth month, the uterus has stretched to about 500 times its prepregnancy size! Its weight increases, starting from a couple of ounces to more than 2 pounds. After pregnancy, the uterus returns to its original size. The muscles and ligaments are incredibly strong and elastic.

## YOUR POSTPARTUM BODY

While your body has achieved this incredible feat (way to go mama!), it has changed and, frankly, based on my personal and professional experience over the past 20 years, this aspect of the postpartum journey has been neglected severely.

> 66 When I was training for a marathon years after having my last child, I started having severe knee pain. When I went to physical therapy, they actually told me it was from my hip. Through weeks of physical therapy, I learned that my pregnancies, deliveries, how I carried my babies on my hip all affected my pelvic alignment, which was causing much of the pain while running. I had no idea that my body was still feeling the effects 5 years later! 99

### *Pelvic Floor*

Your body will naturally change both during the pregnancy as well as after your delivery. That's not surprising. Whether it's your first pregnancy or third, the physicality of what your body is doing will have an effect after you deliver. Your pelvic floor is directly affected during pregnancy, through your delivery, and in your postpartum period.

What is a pelvic floor? The pelvic floor is a dome-shaped muscle that separates the pelvic cavity from the perineal region below. The pelvic cavity encloses the bladder, intestines, and uterus in females. The pelvic floor muscles essentially support all of these major organs. The urethra, vagina, and anus all pass through these pelvic floor muscles. During pregnancy, there will be a shift that will not only affect your muscles, nerves, and ligaments, but also your pelvis, which consists of various bones (hip, sacrum, coccyx). Your pelvis not only supports the weight of the upper body, but also serves as an attachment site for these muscles and ligaments.

### Sciatica

While you may have mild aches and discomfort during your pregnancy, other symptoms can occur as well. Sciatica is one example. I had sciatica during my second pregnancy. It was a sharp pain running down my left leg, which caused me to clunk my foot down when I walked. Unfortunately, back then, no physician or physical therapist wanted to touch a pregnant woman for fear of hurting her or the fetus.

### Incontinence

Some women experience problems related to incontinence during pregnancy or after delivery (vaginal or cesarean) that can lead to a loss of voluntary control of urination and/or defecation. Some of you may be horrified, while others may have experienced it themselves or know someone who has. What I found doing my research is that while this issue has started gaining attention over the past 5 years, there is still little information accessible to pregnant and postpartum women. Even now, physicians and other health care providers who work with pregnant women and postpartum mothers have little to no training about incontinence and are unable to help as they may be unaware of these issues and available resources.

In my 40s, I began to run a lot, like 50 to 75 miles a month. I ran because the exercise benefited my health as well as my mind by relieving stress. It made me feel great. When I began training for another half-marathon, my knee started to hurt. But contrary to years past, I was worried, and I actually decided to get it checked out. After an examination, the physical therapist told me that the problem wasn't my knee; the pain was originating from my hip and pelvis. She told me that carrying 3 children to full-term, in addition to the terrible posture I developed during those years of propping my right hip out to carry my children didn't help. This was the first time, after 3 kids, that I had ever heard of this. After hearing her explanation, the connection made complete sense.

### Episiotomy Pain

Fast-forward 3 years. While I was working more and more with postpartum mothers, the mothers of the babies I was seeing asked me questions about the changes in their own bodies. They asked me about their episiotomy pain. Mamas asked me about their incisions that weren't healing. Some mothers in my office had difficulty sitting down because of horrible tears that occurred during delivery. Based on my own experiences plus what I witnessed in my own practice, I realized that moms' physical changes and healing of their bodies needed to be addressed. I needed to learn more so mamas could receive the help they needed for their physical discomfort and pain.

One mom said, "I thought it was just the normal issues after having a baby. It took me almost 2 years to feel normal." Like this woman, many mothers ignore these issues because their focus is on the newborn and the growing needs of their families. Talking to friends, colleagues, and mothers in my practice, I realized that paying attention to the physical changes that affect the pelvic floor is important in the immediate postpartum period, but it is also important to *prevent* issues from developing later on that will affect our bodies.

Don't just take my word for it. Research shows that up to 80% of women who have a vaginal delivery will experience tearing of the pelvic skin and muscles, causing incontinence in 10%. Also, while the stress of a vaginal delivery can increase the risk of pelvic floor dysfunction, it does not always happen in the immediate postpartum period but can occur years, even decades after delivery. As the muscles weaken during pregnancy and the stress of delivery, the pelvic floor can prolapse, which can cause a drop of the organs within your pelvic cavity, specifically the bladder, uterus, vagina, small bowel, and rectum. Subsequently, this can cause you pain, weakness, and incontinence.

Based on my own experience as well as my observations of new moms experiencing pain and discomfort months and even years after delivery, I've come to realize that the postpartum period—the fourth trimester—must incorporate mom's physical health. Specifically, the pelvic area must be part of the discussion as so many mamas experience pain and discomfort as a result of changes in their pelvic floor.

I still remember the "advice" I received as I was leaving the hospital with my newborn in 2002. After checking the car seat and rolling the baby and me to the parking lot in a wheelchair, the nurse told me, "Don't have sex for 6 weeks." As if I was even thinking about intimacy with my husband. So, yes, this was the extent of the advice we received on this topic 10 to 15 years ago.

Unfortunately, because of the lack of information and proper advice, women usually think that this is just how it's supposed to be. Or mamas may feel they don't have the time to discuss this with their obstetrician during the postpartum visit. And let's face it. Some mamas may be embarrassed talking about this topic and are too afraid to bring it up with the doctor during the postpartum visit. Even when they do ask about it, women may find their concerns brushed off because many in the medical community lack information. This reinforces their feelings that the problem is just something they have to deal with and get through.

## ADVOCATE FOR YOUR HEALTH

Now that I've described everything that happens to your body with pregnancy and childbirth as well as what *can* happen, you're probably thinking, *why* is she telling me this? To worry me more? No, it isn't to scare you. I want you to be aware of these issues so you can empower yourself to ask questions and advocate for your physical health. I want you to realize when that pain and discomfort is not *just* because you had a baby. I want you to understand that this is not normal, and you don't have to just get through it. By empowering yourself with this knowledge, you can ask questions and hopefully find the help you need.

## Pelvic Floor Physical Therapy

So where can you find this help? Everyone reading this has probably heard of physical therapy. I have had physical therapy multiple times for my knee and hip issues (much of which came about after 3 babies) while training for my races. But have you heard about *pelvic floor therapy*? Yes, this is a real thing and it is exactly what it sounds like. Some physical therapists are specially trained in pelvic floor therapy. Thankfully, it is an emerging specialty and continues to grow. Speaking with the pelvic floor specialists in my area and conducting my own research, I have learned and continue to learn so much. Studies show that pelvic floor therapy after giving birth will not only address issues in the immediate postpartum period, but it can prevent long-term problems. Even if you are planning on having more kids/multiple pregnancies, I encourage you to undergo pelvic floor therapy after *each* delivery once your obstetrician gives you the OK. Don't wait (like I did) until after your last pregnancy to address these issues.

While many of us are continuing to learn about this therapy and advocating for mothers, some countries are already offering this therapy for women during the postpartum period. For instance, in France, pelvic physical therapy is a standard part of postpartum care. The obstetrician will prescribe anywhere from 10 to 20 sessions of pelvic physical therapy. An added bonus is that these sessions are part of the postpartum care package that is covered by the governmental health care plan.

Because pelvic floor therapy is still considered a new practice in the United States, not all insurance plans cover it, or you may have to pay extra out-of-network costs. What is promising, however, is that more and more physicians and physical therapists in the United States understand the importance of pelvic floor therapy for postpartum mothers.

## Where to Start?

First, talk with your obstetrician and ask for a referral during your postpartum checkup. Also, talk with your friends as they may have some recommendations. Call your insurance provider to find a physical therapist who specializes in pelvic floor therapy.

While it may seem like there are a lot of hoops to jump through, enlist your husband/partner or family member to help you do the research. Often times, speaking to other women/mothers is a helpful way to find providers who are well-trained in pelvic floor physical therapy. And again, I recommend obtaining this information before the baby arrives (see Chapter 4).

Pelvic floor therapists have treated moms with complaints ranging from neck and back pain, sciatica and tailbone pain, to even incontinence with sneezing or jumping. These problems can result from postural changes that occur not only during pregnancy but afterward depending on how you carry, wear, and even nurse your baby.

Even though you may have only minor symptoms, I recommend seeing a pelvic floor therapist before starting your exercise regimen. Your body just went through a transformative experience. Before you start running, doing yoga, cycling, or lifting weights, don't you want to be sure that your pelvic floor is healing properly? I wish I had! My youngest child is in high school, and even as I write this, my lower back still aches after this morning's run.

## What to Expect at the First Visit?

The initial appointment will consist of a thorough intake in which you will be asked about any symptoms you may be having, your level of physical activity prior to and during the pregnancy, and your birth experience. The therapist will help you identify your goals and what you wish to accomplish during these sessions. Your pelvic floor therapist will gently examine the scarring around your vulva, as well as the scar for mamas who had a cesarean delivery. You should also be aware that the therapist will perform an internal pelvic examination during one of the initial sessions.

Also, while the pelvic floor therapist will be working on exercises to stabilize and strengthen your core and pelvic area, she or he will also teach you mindfulness, visualization, and breathing exercises. The mind-body connection is so important, as is recognizing its role in healing and repairing the physical body.

The number of therapy sessions will vary depending on you, your symptoms, and the number of deliveries you've had. However, these therapy sessions take *time*, and for most, if not all, of you, time is a luxury. I am well aware that each and every one of you is juggling a lot. And while I have encouraged you to take things *off* your plate, pelvic floor therapy sessions are something I seriously want you to consider *adding* to your plate. *You*, mama, are the most important piece of this puzzle. You need to care for yourself just as you care for your newborn and everyone else in your household and family. The preventive nature of pelvic floor therapy is vital. I do not want you to put a bandage, so to speak, on these issues that can cause problems months or even years down the road. What's my mantra? *A happy and healthy mama equals a happy and healthy baby.*

## LET'S TALK ABOUT SEX

Many of you, like me, were told to wait 6 weeks before engaging in sexual intercourse. If you are pregnant or a newly postpartum mama, you probably are thinking I'm crazy talking about having sex. Like the issues many women face as a result of pelvic floor dysfunction, sexual activity after giving birth is frequently not discussed. Often, it is taken for granted that sexual activity will resume, and that pain during sex is normal after giving birth. This is not true. Painful intercourse, also known as *dyspareunia*, is genital pain that is persistent or recurrent and can occur before, during, or after sex. I hope some of you are feeling a sense of relief because I am telling you right now mamas, you are not alone. Even though this issue is common, it usually is not talked about.

## *Painful Sex*

Studies show that 50% of women experience painful sex after giving birth (and that's just the women who report their symptoms). Dyspareunia can start at 6 weeks postpartum and continue up to 6 months postpartum—or even longer. Dyspareunia can happen to any postpartum mother, whether she had a natural delivery or cesarean delivery, and it can occur after any or all deliveries. The pain most often occurs during penetration. It can be a result of excessive dryness, which can be exacerbated by breastfeeding because hormonal changes can reduce your natural lubrication. Experts recommend using a water-based lubricant to help with pain as your body heals. If that doesn't work, talk to your obstetrician about a prescription for a topical estrogen cream that can add moisture.

It is also important for you to talk with your partner about the pain and symptoms you are experiencing during sex, so they understand the importance of being gentle during intercourse.

However, persistent pain during intercourse should not be ignored. I don't want you to just get through it while you're clenching your teeth in pain. This needs to be addressed as it can be due to excessive scarring, or it is possible that something didn't heal properly after giving birth. Although this is a sensitive topic and often one that does not get discussed, I want you to know that you are not alone in this. First and foremost, I encourage you to speak with your partner/spouse about how you are feeling. The person with whom you are intimate should listen to your concerns and understand the changes you are going though. And while it may alter certain aspects of your relationship, realize (and tell your partner!) that this is temporary. The goal is for you to get the help you need early on so these issues can be addressed. I know this topic may be difficult for some of you, but just know that communication and honesty are key.

Although you may feel rushed or even embarrassed to talk about this with your physician during the postpartum visit, please mention it. Whether you need a prescription to help with lubrication or a referral to a specialist, it is important to inform your obstetrician about the discomfort you are having.

Ongoing dyspareunia can be the result of issues with your pelvic floor and is another great reason to receive pelvic physical therapy. The muscles and pelvic floor tissue can be injured or weakened during pregnancy and childbirth, and pelvic floor therapy can help strengthen and heal.

### Surgery May Be Needed

In more severe cases, surgery may be warranted. Depending on your pain and physical needs, a surgeon may recommend waiting until you have completed having children. However, if you continue to have severe pain/discomfort, incontinence, or other symptoms described earlier, your physician can refer you to a surgeon who specializes in female pelvic medicine and reproductive surgery. This can be a gynecologist, a urologist, or a urogynecologist. Obtaining this referral doesn't automatically mean you are going to need surgery, but it is important for the surgeon to perform a full evaluation while giving you all the information you need to make an informed decision. Mama, it is important for you to feel empowered and advocate for *yourself*. Information is powerful and will help you decide what is right for you and your physical health.

During the first 6 weeks after giving birth, you will experience afterpains, also known as *involution*. Basically, these are cramps and they can be really painful. During the 9 months of your pregnancy, your uterus expanded to make space for a small human being, and it is now shrinking back to its normal size. The human body is truly amazing, isn't it? These short sharp cramps are not only contracting your uterus, they are also contracting the uterine blood vessels, which helps to prevent blood clots and reduce your postpartum bleeding. My nursing moms will experience more intense cramps, as involution is triggered by oxytocin, also known as the love hormone. Oxytocin is released when the breast/nipple is stimulated by either the baby or a breast pump. As long as you have no contraindication or allergies, you can take ibuprofen for these cramps. I always recommend that you have something in your stomach, even a small snack, so your stomach lining doesn't become irritated by the ibuprofen. There is no risk in taking ibuprofen while breastfeeding as none of it will pass through your breast milk to the baby.

### Contraception

At that postpartum check with your obstetrician, you will be discussing birth control. Before you head into that visit, you will need to consider your fertility goals. This is an important discussion to have with your spouse/partner before the appointment. Do you want to get pregnant again? If so, when? How far apart do you want your children to be? Consider your age, your partner's age, your health, and your stage of life. Discussing these issues with your partner is important when deciding which birth control will be best for you both. Your needs and desires probably have changed over time. What works for you, your lifestyle, your spouse/partner? Your goals after your first baby likely differ from those after your second or third baby. To help you get started, go to Bedsider (https://www.bedsider. org/methods) for up-to-date, evidence-based information that moms can use to compare and contrast methods. Make sure to have an idea of the birth control method you are interested in using and talk to your doctor about which options might work best for you.

Again, going into this appointment with an idea of what you and your family want and need will help you when making this important decision.

Let me add that, for many couples, the responsibility for birth control can fall on the male partner. However, it is important to know what works best for you and your partner in terms of successfully preventing pregnancy. Also, while this may not happen to all women, hormonal birth control may cause vaginal dryness, as vaginal lubrication is linked to estrogen levels in your body. While some studies show changes in libido based on the type of hormonal birth control used, these changes vary greatly based on the type of birth control as well as you, the person. Therefore, talk with your doctor about all of your concerns.

### *For My Breastfeeding Mamas*

For breastfeeding mamas, there are certain things to consider. First, hormonal birth control is not recommended until your breast milk supply is well-established, which is usually around the 4- to 6-week period. The most important thing to consider with hormonal birth control and breastfeeding is estrogen because it can decrease your breast milk supply. Based on the evidence, if you want to use or resume using hormonal birth control for your family planning needs, it is best to wait at least 6 weeks postpartum before starting and/or placement of a hormonal birth control method. Also, progestin-only or lower-dose estrogen hormonal birth control is preferred because of the possible adverse effects of estrogen on breast milk supply.

In many countries, cultures, and religions, breastfeeding is used as a form of birth control. This method is called *lactation amenorrhea method* (LAM). However, to be an effective form of birth control—meaning to prevent a pregnancy—3 specific criteria must be met:

1. Mom must be exclusively or nearly exclusively breastfeeding. If there is some occasional supplementation, it is rare and does not disrupt the frequency of breastfeeding sessions.
2. You must not have had any periods, which is defined as the return of bleeding that occurs after 56 days (2 months) postpartum or any 2 consecutive days of menstrual bleeding.
3. Baby is 6 months or younger, because at 6 months of age, they have often started first foods.

LAM can be used as an initial method of birth control while you are waiting to start another method. Evidence shows that for mothers who are exclusively breastfeeding, it is highly unlikely that they will become pregnant within the first 2 months (56 days), thus allowing moms to delay other forms of birth control for 8 weeks postpartum.

Whether it is based on accessibility, affordability, and/or cultural and religious beliefs, women all over the world use LAM as a form of birth control. For instance, 1 study in Pakistan showed that almost 400 women who were exclusively breastfeeding were counseled about this form of birth control. When used correctly, less than 1% of women became pregnant while breastfeeding during those first 6 months. However, once their menstrual period restarted, this method was no longer effective.

Discussing all your options with your physician is important so you find what works best for you, your baby, your partner, and your life.

# CHAPTER 11

# Ease the Stress of Returning to Work

**WORK**/noun/wərk/: activity involving mental or physical effort done in order to achieve a purpose or result

I remember when my daughter was 5 months old and it was time for me to return to my fellowship program so I could graduate on time. My husband, a physician in the intensive care unit who worked 60 hours a week, was on call most weekends and did not have any paternity leave. Reliable child care that would work for our schedules was essential. We had no relatives who lived close by, so we knew that we would have to leave our baby with a stranger. It was unsettling, and I was both sad and stressed. At one point, I told my husband that I was going to give up my career and stay home with our new baby. So what if I didn't finish my training? Like so many women, I had so much mom guilt. The opinions of some did not help this already difficult decision, and my own feelings were overwhelming. My husband was extremely supportive, but in order for me to finish my medical training, I had to go back to work. Thankfully, our family and friends told me that I needed to go back, that it would be good for both the baby and me. I knew I wanted my career, but I felt guilty about leaving my baby.

Despite what your family unit looks like, regardless of how long you stay home after having your baby, or how much support you will have once you are home, deciding who is going to care for your infant once you return to school or work is an agonizing decision. What I learned, based on my own experience plus seeing young women I work with struggle with this decision, is that you need to start thinking about child care and discussing it with your spouse/partner early, ideally before the baby arrives.

Planning for child care is one of the most important aspects of the postpartum period, but new parents are woefully unprepared. This is not to say it is anyone's fault; we are caught up in the initial baby stages, enjoying the baby, attempting to breastfeed, trying to survive many sleepless nights, and enjoying the time we have at home with our newborn. Also, in many areas, accessible and affordable child care is not easy to find. Although there are options, researching what works for you, the baby, and your family does take time. Considering all your options before the baby arrives and figuring out what will best meet your and your partner's needs will help alleviate stress and allow you to spend your maternity leave bonding with your baby.

## FIGURING OUT YOUR CHILD CARE OPTIONS

So mama, what are your options for child care? Whether it's a family member, friend, child care center, nanny, or long-term au pair, first and foremost, you and your partner need to sit down and decide what will work best for both of you.

## *Things to Consider*

What are your and your partner's work hours? How early do you have to leave the house? How late do you work? Do you both work Monday through Friday, or will there be weekend hours? Will you need help throughout the day or maybe just a few hours in the morning? Don't forget about your commute. Do you live in an area where traffic is unpredictable? Will an employer offer any flexibility? Is working remotely from home an option? It will be helpful for you and your partner to map out your needs as you begin researching child care options.

Now that you have figured out the days and hours you need someone to care for your baby, you can start looking at your options. Do you want more than a babysitter? Will it be helpful to have someone do laundry, clean a bit, and even prepare dinner for your family? Remember, in those early months your baby will be napping much of the day.

## *What Is Your Comfort Level?*

Are you comfortable having someone in your home with your infant versus bringing your baby to a group setting with multiple children and numerous child care providers? It is also important to consider your baby's exposure to other children, especially during those winter months.

What happens if your child care provider takes a sick day or goes on vacation? What if your child becomes sick and cannot go to a group setting? Is your job/workplace flexible or do you have to consider a back-up child care plan?

You may also need to consider the layout of your home and your living space. Are you in a home that can accommodate another person or in a smaller apartment where space may be an issue?

You might also need to consider the difference between employing a stranger and having a family member or friend provide child care. Sometimes, if child care is viewed as helping versus employment, reliability may be an issue if your family member or friend has other commitments, such as family, work, or travel. Also, approaching a family member or friend with a job description and specific duties can be a bit difficult.

## LET'S TAKE A CLOSER LOOK AT YOUR OPTIONS

### Nanny

A nanny is a child care provider who comes into your home. There can be flexibility regarding the number of days and hours. If you don't need a full-time nanny, families have been known to share a nanny so this person will have full-time employment while meeting the needs of multiple families. How will you pay this person (hourly, daily, monthly salary)? Will you provide benefits, such as sick time and vacation pay? Will you be paying social security tax and income taxes? Deciding this at the outset is important to avoid confusion or hurt feelings. I recommend a trial period to make sure that this person works for your baby and family, and that your family is a good fit for the nanny. Also, it is important to lay out your expectations in the beginning, whether that means a feeding and napping schedule for your baby, laundering the baby's clothes, doing some light housekeeping, and even prepping dinner. The work environment is changing drastically, and few of us work from 9 to 5. Will your nanny be able to accommodate your schedule—whether that is working from home or working late nights or even weekends—and be flexible?

A live-in nanny is also an option. When I lived in New York City, within our Indian community, many families hired a nanny who lived with them 5 days a week and then had the weekend off. For many friends and family, this worked well because they had the space, had help at night, and did not feel they had to rush home from work. However, you have to be comfortable with someone living in your home—and have that space.

For us, having a nanny during the day worked best for both of our hectic work schedules. We did not have the space in our apartment or feel comfortable having someone live with us. However, with our busy medical careers, the flexibility a nanny gave us was ideal. Our first nanny also did the baby's laundry and some light cleaning and even cooked fresh Indian food for us! Putting my daughter in child care was not an option for my family as we were required to be at the center by 6 pm to pick her up; if we were late, they would start charging us added fees in 15-minute increments. Our hours were always unpredictable, plus contending with New York City traffic made it highly unlikely that one of us could get to the child care center by 6 pm. So hiring a nanny was our best option. For me, it was a bonus not having to awaken and dress the baby in those early mornings and then sit in traffic.

> 66 I interviewed nannies the month before I was going back to work. This was my first baby, we had no family nearby, and my husband's schedule was worse than mine. I look back now and realize how thankful I am that my mom was there for the interviews with me. I was so nervous. I wasn't sure if I was asking the right questions or really hearing what she was saying. I had already thought about quitting since I was so sad about leaving my daughter with a stranger. 99

## Cultural Sensitivity When it Comes to Child Care

Child care should go hand in hand with what happens at home. Young children need to feel good about where they come from. To feel secure, babies need to have the same experiences at home that they do when they are in someone's care. If your child is attending a child care center, are there certain things he or she should or should not have based on cultural or religious beliefs? Will certain dietary restrictions be accommodated, such as not eating meat or other foods that are not allowed based on religious beliefs? This is important to consider when researching outside child care settings to make sure they can accommodate your requests and the child's needs.

For many of us from different countries and cultures, our babies or toddlers will be exposed to different languages as they enter child care. I always encourage the parents of my patients in the United States to maintain their mother tongue in the home because the child will be exposed to and learn English in child care. It is truly a gift to be bilingual at such a young age.

Culture is also important to consider when someone is coming into your home. If the caregiver is a grandparent or other family member, many times the cultural customs and language will overlap with what your child is already exposed to in the home. But this may not be the case when hiring a nanny or an au pair. Make sure that the person coming into your home understands and honors your customs and beliefs. For instance, everyone who enters my home must take off their shoes before walking through the house. Even now, all of my kids' friends know that their sneakers or flip flops come off at the Sriraman house! One of the nannies we interviewed was from India and spoke my language, but she couldn't speak English. I was worried whether she would be able to call 911 and communicate in an emergency. Also, my husband, who is from a different part of India, speaks an entirely different language. Although she was lovely, we couldn't hire her because she and my husband weren't able to communicate.

Culture is the fundamental building block of identity, and honoring diversity strengthens relationships with parents and those taking care of our children.

## Au Pairs

Many companies, including international companies, place young women and men in homes as au pairs. The au pair has the opportunity to live in another country and become more proficient in another language. An au pair lessens the burden for many families who have more varied working hours. However, au pairs are limited in the number of hours they can work per week. There is also a requirement that au pairs have their own room and often a mode of transportation. Depending on the age of the child(ren), the au pair will be transporting them, and if your children are school-aged, the au pair often attends classes at the local college to enhance his or her education. Again, every company is a bit different, so it is important to verify the requirements.

> 66 As a teacher, I have to be at school by 7 am and since my husband travels for work 4 days a week, there is no one at home with my children in those early morning hours. An au pair worked well for our family since she was able to get them on the bus and be home when they came home. My kids cried at the end of the year when she had to return to Germany. 99

A friend of mine, who was widowed with children, was a general surgeon who could be called to the hospital at all hours, day or night. For her, a male au pair worked well as he acted like an older brother to her sons.

## Child Care

Whether it is at another person's home, a regulated child care facility, or a center at your workplace, your baby will be with other infants/children in a group setting. You will take your child to this location along with the items needed for that day, such as diapers, breast milk or formula, a change of clothes, and a pacifier. Be sure to ask your child care provider if you need to supply baby food or table food once your baby starts eating solids. Many child care centers are only open on weekdays and have specific hours for drop-off and pickup. If the child care facility is close to your work or even affiliated with your job, you may have the opportunity to see your baby during the workday to hold, play with, and even nurse directly (forgoing the need to pump at that time).

Your baby will be exposed to other children and different child care providers depending on the child's age. Does the facility have activities during the day? Do the children go outside to play? What procedures are in place to ensure your baby's safety as people enter and exit the building? These are important questions to ask. It is also essential to find out their policy for when your child is sick. Usually, babies with a fever, rash, or diarrhea must be fever and symptom free for 24 hours before they can return to child care. Also, be sure to find out if the child care facility requires a note from your pediatrician before allowing the baby to return to child care to minimize the spread of illness.

## THINGS TO CONSIDER

One thing to remember is that children are like petri dishes. They're cute, but they carry and transmit lots and lots of germs. In the winter, they will have coughs, colds, and runny noses—I am around this all day. So, while it may be frightening at first, your baby's immune system is bolstered by being exposed to other children.

Please keep in mind that depending on where you live, some child care centers have long waiting lists, and you will have to put your name on that list while you are pregnant! It may be that the area doesn't have many child care providers, or if you live in a larger city, the demand for good child care is high.

For many of my friends, child care worked out well. They felt comfortable that their children would be in a group setting, being monitored by different adults while interacting with other

> 66 My twins really enjoy child care. They are around other toddlers their age and learn so much from the teachers. I actually come home early from work a few days a week, run errands, clean up the house, and then go pick them up. I love having those extra hours to myself while they are at the child care center so I can get things done. 99

children their age. Depending on their work schedules, one parent would drop off the child in the morning while the other parent, who finished the work day earlier, picked up the child before the facility closed, and they didn't need weekend coverage.

It is normal to feel confused or overwhelmed. For me, the whole process of finding child care while trying to get into back-to-work mode and managing my own feelings was overwhelming. But I am here to tell you that the more you can prepare for these situations, and the earlier you start, the more relaxed you will feel. I promise.

Where do you start? First, talk with your partner and decide what help you will need and when you will need it. Sometimes, start-ing at this point will help you narrow down your choices. Mamas, do not minimize the power of your network. Whether you talk to neighbors, other moms, friends with children, or colleagues, ask what they are doing for child care. Word-of-mouth is extremely powerful. When we relocated to a new state where we had just one friend in our small city, I was blessed (and still am) to have found our current nanny through another mom I met at my son's preschool. Seriously, 411 has nothing on us mamas! Start researching 2 to 3 months before you'll need child care to begin. If you can start looking at options while you are pregnant, please do so. However, if you plan to have an extended maternity leave, depending on the options available to you, child care providers may not meet with you if your start date is too far in the future. But starting to research child care providers and contacting them before you deliver will give you enough time to review your child-care options without feeling rushed or stressed.

A few things I recommend as you research options and interview individuals or centers. Ask for references and call them! This is so important for you to feel comfortable leaving your child with a person who is safe. Also, ask the child care providers if they are trained in infant/child cardiopulmonary resuscitation (CPR). As this may not be the case for someone coming into your home, paying for your child care provider to receive CPR training is well worth the money.

If possible, it may be beneficial to have another mother (friend, sister, mother) conduct the interviews and/or tour the child care centers with you. While my husband was aware, he had no earthly clue what to look for or ask potential nannies. Frankly, mamas have a sixth sense—call it a Spidey-sense if you will—about the nuances of what we need for our family and our baby. However, as a new mom, you may be quite anxious and forget to ask key questions, which is why it can be helpful to have another mother, including older female family members, with you during the interview.

When I went back to work that first week, my husband took time off so I would be less anxious returning to my clinical work environment and not have to worry about a new person watching my baby. During the second week, I was fortunate that my mother could stay with us, and even though she wasn't taking care of the baby, she was in the apartment being my eyes while the new nanny was with my baby. Do what works best for you to minimize the distress of leaving your baby for the first time. It will be stressful and you may be sad, but I hope these strategies will help minimize your feelings of worry and sadness.

## Key Questions to Consider if You Hire Someone

Payment: What will be the method of payment? Will you be providing benefits? Will you pay on an hourly basis or make a lump sum payment?

Vacation: Will you offer vacation time? If so, will it be paid? How much time will be allowed?

Sick Time: Will you provide sick time? What about any family emergencies the child care provider might have?

Transportation: If the child care provider will be responsible for driving your kids around, will you provide reimbursement for gas?

Hours: Will the hours be consistent or varied? Might these change?

Responsibilities: Will you require the child care provider to do light cleaning or laundry or prepare meals?

Visitors: Will the child care provider be allowed to have visitors over? Will you need to establish rules?

Driving: Will the child care provider be required to drive your child around? If so, will you need to lend a car with a car seat?

## MATERNITY LEAVE

Let's talk maternity leave. For those of you who live outside the United States, I am immensely envious of the maternity leave and family friendly policies many countries have for mothers (and fathers) in the immediate postpartum period.

Over the past 20 years, women have made up anywhere between 50% and 60% of the US labor workforce. Yes, at least half of American workers are women, many of whom are mothers. In 2020, 71% of working women were mothers. More than 75% of working mothers have children aged 6 to 17, 65% of working mothers have kids who are younger than 6, and 63% of working moms have children who are younger than 3 years. Women, especially mothers, are the fastest growing segment of the workforce.

Working outside the home is a choice for many women and some, like me, love our careers and want to continue working. However, for many mothers, going back to work is a financial necessity.

Sadly, paid family medical leave in the United States is nonexistent. While it has been getting more traction in the media and is being discussed in the political realm in terms of infrastructure to help the country's economy, we are still light-years behind. I have colleagues who come back 6 weeks after a cesarean delivery to a grueling on-call schedule. I see moms in my practice who work in hourly wage jobs and are required to return to work only 2 weeks after giving birth! Even putting aside the emotional and mental aspects of the postpartum period, have people forgotten that we just nourished another human being for 9 months and then expelled him or her from our bodies?

In the United States, if you receive paid maternity leave, it is often not more than 6 weeks. Those of us in the medical field are required to use our vacation time. Depending on the job, many women will not receive any paid maternity leave, so during the time they are not working after giving birth, these mothers are not making any money and, in fact, are losing wages. While some states and companies provide maternity leave, it is often not required. Some women I know have applied for unpaid time off under the Family and Medical Leave Act or filed for short-term disability, which involves a lot of paperwork. Neither is ideal and frankly it just adds to our stress as we figure out what works for us economically while deciphering coverage plans and wading through paperwork. Unfortunately, the United States is 1 of only 5 countries in the United Nations that does not provide paid maternity leave. The other 4 countries are developing nations that have much worse economies than the United States. I'm talking a 100-fold difference in gross domestic product.

Depending on your family's personal and financial needs, discussing maternity leave with your employer *while* you are pregnant is essential to avoid surprises. If you are a contracted employee, make sure maternity leave is in your contract. For example, I had an employer who threatened to pull my health insurance because I was taking "extra time off" after being placed on bed rest. For many women, this can feel like a daunting task, but it is important to speak with your employer early on so you know all your options and can plan accordingly.

## FOR MY BREASTFEEDING MAMAS, HOW CAN YOU PREPARE?

Going back to work as a breastfeeding mother is an issue of much importance, but few if any mothers receive the guidance they need. In my breastfeeding telehealth practice, moms often set up appointments to discuss back-to-work issues a few weeks beforehand. First of all, I don't want you trying out your new pump on the first day of work! I counsel all my mothers to start pumping 3 to 4 weeks prior to your return date. This gives you time to familiarize yourself with the pump, including the settings and how to dismantle and wash it. You also need to figure out what type of bra you will need. Fortunately, there are so many options out there that I didn't have 15 years ago. There are specialized bras that incorporate your pump flanges, which allows you to do hands-free pumping! Some moms even pump while they drive—amazing, right? There are also portable pumps that fit inside your bra; they are almost silent, which allows you to pump while you work. I know many surgeons who use these portable pumps because they may go hours without a break.

> 66 I'm not even going to start breastfeeding, except the colostrum. I'll give the baby that in the hospital. I am only home for 6 weeks, but once I go back to work, I will not be able to pump. There is no dedicated space and the door to my classroom has windows so I have no privacy. So why even bother starting? 99

Moms, when you start pumping to build up your supply, I want you to start slowly to avoid becoming overwhelmed. Your body makes the most milk in the early morning hours. Many of you wake up for that early morning nursing session with extremely heavy breasts, with breast milk leaking onto your t-shirt and sometimes even the bedsheets. If possible, after that early morning nursing session, hand your baby to another person, who can burp the baby, change the diaper, and have a snuggle session with the baby. And you start pumping. Pumping during the early morning will yield the most milk, thereby allowing you to start building your supply.

At work, plan for 1 pumping session at least every 3 to 4 hours to maintain your milk supply. Depending on your work schedule, if you nurse before leaving home and immediately when you arrive home, you may only have to pump once or twice at work. Also, keep in mind that your breasts will tell you when it's time to pump. Although pumping every 3 to 4 hours is ideal to maintain your milk supply, mothers who have smaller breasts and/or a larger supply may need to pump more frequently.

> **66** While I was still breastfeeding my second child, I tried my best to pump at work. Luckily, I had an office with a door that locked so I had some privacy. But while I pumped, I didn't have those 15 to 20 minutes to just relax, which affected my let-down and supply. After only about 5 to 10 minutes, a staff member would start pounding on my door, telling me that my patients were waiting for me. Needless to say, my supply dropped and I stopped pumping. I felt terrible, but I continued to nurse the baby before and after work. **99**

Where are you going to pump? Based on the Affordable Care Act of 2010, you should *not*, let me repeat, *not* be pumping in a bathroom. Would you eat your lunch while sitting on the toilet? Of course not, so why should your baby's lunch be prepared there? By law, you should have a private space where you can lock the door and breastfeed. If there is a sink close by, that is ideal because it is important to wash and rinse the pump parts before you store them. Where will you store your pumped milk? Do you have access to a small refrigerator or will you need to store your milk in a small cooler? Your response may depend, at least in part, on your comfort level as you may not want your breast milk (or your colleagues') stored in a refrigerator in a common work area.

When you come home from work mamas, I want you to hand off the breast pump to your partner or a child care provider if you have someone caring for the baby in your home. While you label the breast milk pumped at work, the other person can wash the pump flanges or put them into the dishwasher. Then I want you to snuggle with your baby and nurse if the baby is hungry. Relax and put up your feet and just enjoy being home with your baby in your arms. Got it? All the other stuff can wait.

### Storing Your Breast Milk

So you're being a rock star and pumping milk at work. How do you safely store it and for how long? The stories I hear from mothers regarding what they've been told about breast milk storage still shock me. One mom said, "The nurse in the hospital told me that I couldn't combine the pumped milk from 9 am with the pumped milk from noon, so since the baby was only taking 2 ounces, I had to throw an ounce down the drain after each pumping session." Understandably, she became emotional and we both began to cry. Yes, I know it's the doctor's office, but that story broke my heart.

Remember, breast milk is liquid gold for your baby. With all of its benefits (discussed in Chapter 7), are you surprised? Thus, I do not want anyone reading this book to discard breast milk down the drain. What are the guidelines? I like to use the Rule of 4s—super easy for my mamas and me to remember.

## Remember the Rule of 4s for Storing Breast Milk

Freshly expressed breast milk can be stored at room temperature for up to **4** hours.

Freshly expressed breast milk can be stored in a refrigerator for **4** days.

Reminder: When placed in the refrigerator or freezer, breast milk should be stored toward the back, not in the door, because it is exposed to room temperature every time you open the door. Make sure to write the date you pumped the breast milk on the outside of the bag so you know when it expires.

(For more information, please see Human Milk Storage Guidelines on page 73.)

Once frozen breast milk is taken out of the freezer and thaws, it cannot be refrozen. So even if you pump a large amount at work, when you come home, I recommend freezing the expressed breast milk in 2- to 4-ounce aliquots so it will not be wasted once it's taken out of the freezer. When filling a container with expressed breast milk, be sure to leave space at the top to allow for expansion with freezing.

Previously frozen milk may be kept in the refrigerator for up to 24 hours after it has thawed. If your baby does not finish the milk at one feeding, it is considered safe to refrigerate the milk and offer it within 2 to 3 hours before discarding it.

You can thaw frozen milk slowly by putting it in the refrigerator the night before; it will take approximately 12 hours to thaw. If you need to thaw it more quickly, hold the container under warm running water.

To warm up expressed breast milk, place it under running water or use a bottle warmer. Never microwave your breast milk for 2 reasons: (1) it will kill many of the protective antibodies in the breast milk and (2) microwaving any milk (formula included) can produce hot pockets within the bottle that can cause a thermal burn in your baby's mouth.

For my pumping mamas, you will notice how the milk forms layers after it has been sitting in your refrigerator. The cream will rise to the top of the milk during storage. (For more information on the importance of foremilk and hindmilk, see Chapter 7.) While you do not want to shake the bottle, you should gently swirl the expressed milk to mix the components, and always check the temperature of the milk before offering it to the baby.

If you are pumping at different times during the day, you can combine the pumped amounts into 1 container at the end of that day.

I used to pump directly into a bottle because it was easier to cap and close at work. Once I got home, I poured the pumped breast milk into 3- to 4-ounce aliquots. I didn't want to fuss with storage bags at work when I was already feeling rushed. The pump that I used with all 3 of my kids had standard bottles that were compatible with the pump. So, mamas, while you are figuring out your pumping regimen as you prepare to return to work, try out different things to see what works best for you. Having your pumping situation sorted out, including talking with your employer, before returning to work will make the transition much easier.

Remember to label your expressed breast milk with the date and time it was pumped. This will help you and others caring for and feeding the baby identify which milk to use, as you want to use the older containers first so the milk doesn't expire.

Because other people in my household were feeding my babies expressed milk, I was fiercely protective of the breast milk I stored in both the refrigerator and the freezer. Why wouldn't I be, right? It takes a lot of work! What I recommend to all my moms and their partners is to put up a sign outlining the storage guidelines for the breast milk in the refrigerator and freezer, with clear instructions on which bags to use first. This was helpful for my husband and nanny as they didn't have to guess which milk to use while I was at work or away at a conference. Be sure to place a sign on each area of storage (eg, the refrigerator in the kitchen, the freezer in your garage). (Please find a sample breast milk storage guidelines sign on my website at NatashaMomMD.com.)

For my mamas who keep a large supply of breast milk in their freezers, please consider donating some of it to a HMBANA (Human Milk Banking Association of North America) milk bank. These milk banks have regulations and guidelines so that donated breast milk can be pasteurized and used for preterm infants in the neonatal intensive care unit. While breast milk is so important for all our babies, the benefits for preterm infants are even greater, and donated breast milk can help survival rates. I have had physician trainees who donated their milk to our local milk bank because they were relocating to another part of the country and didn't want their breast milk to go to waste. You can find a milk bank anywhere in the world at www. hmbana.org/find-a-milk-bank/.

> 66 I was getting penalized at work for taking time to pump breast milk. So you know what I did? I started keeping track of everyone who left their desk to go out and smoke and how long they were outside. And of course, they weren't getting their pay docked. After a week, I took that information to my boss who suddenly allowed me to take the time to pump twice during my workday. 99

This story came from a mom I interviewed as part of a research project. I was so impressed and applauded her ingenuity. However, it shouldn't be that hard for mothers to do something for our baby's health and well-being. Thankfully, because of federal law, you have rights when it comes to pumping at work without repercussions. I am not saying that it will always be easy, and you may have to continue to advocate for yourself, but you have the law behind you. In 2010, the Affordable Care Act, Section 4207, added a provision to protect moms pumping in the workplace.

## Affordable Care Act

SEC. 4207. Reasonable Break Time for Nursing Mothers

Section 7 of the Fair Labor Standards Act of 1938 (29 U.S.C. 207) is amended by adding at the end the following:

(1) An employer shall provide—"(A) a reasonable break time for an employee to express breast milk for her nursing child for 1 year after the child's birth each time such employee has need to express the milk; and

"(B) a place, other than a bathroom, that is shielded from view and free from intrusion from coworkers and the public, which may be used by an employee to express breast milk.

## SUPPORTING BREASTFEEDING MOTHERS

In 2011, the Surgeon General recognized the importance of supporting breastfeeding mothers in the workplace. Breastfeeding not only helped mothers and babies, but companies that had lactation support programs in place had higher retention rates, better morale, less illness, and lower health expenses for their companies.

Many insurance companies cover breast pumps, so in your third trimester, be sure to contact your health insurance company so it can deliver the breast pump directly to your home. Additionally, breast pumps and other supplies that assist lactation are considered part of medical care. As of 2010, the Internal Revenue Service deemed that any supplies that assist with lactation qualify for tax breaks and/or money can be used from your employer-sponsored flexible spending account. Again, there may be some variation depending on your employer and your state, so I encourage you or your partner to look into this.

When you pump at work, you want privacy so you can relax and not be disturbed. Many mothers and employers have gotten creative with dedicated space and signs that give pumping moms privacy. A few of these names are Nursing Nook, Baby's Lunch Room, and Infant Fueling Station. Even a sign that just says "lactation room" helps support nursing mothers in the workplace.

Remember mamas, during your third trimester, before you begin your official maternity leave, make an appointment with your employer or your human resources representative. While you are discussing your maternity leave, it is also important to tell your employer what you will need once you return to work. That way, you will be on the same page, and the company will have time to prepare accordingly. You will also feel less stressed. Believe me, establishing this before delivery will help you manage some of the stress and worry you may feel returning to work.

## Tips and Tricks to Prepare Yourself for Your First Day Back at Work

- Do you think you will need a trial run on your first day back? Perhaps start with a half day.

- Prepare for your first day back by packing everything you need the day before.

- Do you have a list of emergency contacts and phone numbers for the person watching your baby?

- Remember to leave a to-do list for the person who will be staying home with your baby.

- Make sure to check with your child care facility that they have all your contact information.

- Make sure to pack your baby's child care bag with all the necessities the night before to make sure you don't forget anything that morning.

- Return to work on a Thursday so you don't have to get through a full week the first week back.

# CHAPTER 12

# Reconnecting With Your Partner

**PARTNER**/noun/ˈpärtnər/: either member of a married couple or of an established unmarried couple

I identify as cisgender (she/her/hers). I have been married to my husband for 24 years. My experience as a cisgender female in a heterosexual marriage will be different from that of many of you. To honor the diversity in everyone's relationships, I will use various terms for inclusivity.

Once you have a baby, your marriage, your relationship with your partner *will* change. That is not to say it will get better or worse; it will just be different. I'm telling you this because sometimes it may be hard to accept that change in your relationship.

## STORY TIME

Let me tell you a story about when my oldest child was just a month old. My husband and I always went to this tiny Italian bistro to celebrate our wedding anniversary each year. We had started going to this bistro before we had kids and wanted to keep this tradition. The owners knew us well and were always willing to work to seat us regardless of how busy they were. They were thrilled when we told them I was pregnant and they knew that eventually we would be coming in with our newborn. I was so excited to be getting out of the house and going on our first family outing. I showered, pumped a bottle, and somehow fit my lactating breasts into a sundress. I went through my daughter's new outfits and picked out the cutest one. Finally, we were ready to go. I buckled my baby into her car seat. Instantly, she began to cry. And cry. And cry. I was beside myself because no matter what I tried, she wouldn't stop crying. My husband kept calm, called the restaurant, and was told it would be no problem if we were running late. I became so stressed out because I knew the 45-minute drive would only make her, and me, feel worse.

In the end, I was so upset I decided not to go out. Of course, the night turned out fine. We ordered takeout from another restaurant near home and ate in together. Looking back at the big picture, it was fine. The 3 of us were together, and that made me feel good. However, at the same time, it wasn't fine. I felt sad and defeated, as if I had lost something. As expected, our marriage post-baby looked very different from our pre-baby days. Some of you reading this may think how silly and selfish she is. But others may understand what I was feeling at that point.

Many of you may have had a similar experience or felt the same way, and guess what? It's OK to feel guilty, you may even feel resentment. Although you love and cherish this new baby of yours, it is OK to acknowledge that you've lost some freedom, and even feel sad about it. While you have gained something, you may also feel that you have lost something. Something that you may have taken for granted before the baby. Being able to rush out to meet a friend, go out to dinner with your spouse, or go for a quick workout at the gym. There is a loss of a certain sense of freedom that you shared as a couple. Although it may be tough to accept at first, I promise you that the sense of freedom is not gone. Just changed.

It is important for moms to share these stories, these feelings of sadness and guilt that go along with losing a certain sense of independence. As new mothers, we often are expected to be overjoyed, grateful, and happy all the time. But that is not the reality. By talking about it (like I just did), we normalize these feelings. Instead of feeling shame or believing that your feelings are wrong, by sharing our stories we are making it OK to feel this way.

> 66 My mom and dad kicked us out of the house to babysit my 2-month old daughter. She told me how easy it is to lose focus on your marriage/relationship. But she reminded me that when your kids grow up and leave the house, you want to have something still there instead of just staring at each other in 18 years figuring out who that person is. 99

I wish I could have included the picture from that night. My husband in a black suit and me in a red top (the only one that could contain my large breasts!). It was our first night out, away from our baby for the first time. I was going out on a date with my husband and another couple for an adults only dinner and drinks. For the first time in months, I didn't need to worry about a car seat, a stroller, or a crying baby. You know what? I was really nervous, sad, and a little scared. But like I said, I had no choice; my mother and my husband were going to get me out that door for a break.

## YOU ARE NOT THE SOLE PROVIDER

In Chapter 5, I explained how important it is to involve your partner in all aspects of the postpartum period, whether it's feeding the newborn so you can sleep, taking the siblings to the park, or cooking and cleaning. It is important to establish early on that you are not the sole caregiver for the baby and any siblings, and you are not the only one responsible for maintaining the house. While you may be the sole source of nutrition for the baby (if you're breastfeeding), that doesn't mean you're in charge of everything else.

Let your partner know how you feel. What is that one thing you miss most and don't want to give up? What would you like to do that does not involve your baby, that will make you feel happy and less stressed and even recharge your batteries? For me, it was working out again once my obstetrician gave me the OK. For some, it may be spending time with a close friend. Or having time to yourself to read, watch a show, or maybe cook a gourmet meal. Whatever it is, convey this to your partner. Look at your schedules and try to coordinate a time just for yourself. Maybe nurse your baby and then hand the baby to your spouse so you can go work out or meet a friend. Or ask your partner to take the baby (along with any older children) out for a walk so you can have time to yourself in the house. If this is not an option for you, consider asking a friend or a relative or hiring a babysitter for a few hours. Either way, communicate your needs to your partner, a family member, or a friend.

### Your Partner's Feelings

It is important to realize that for our husbands/partners, there is also a change. While it may seem silly, they may feel helpless. I mean you just birthed a human being, right! They may be trying to figure out where they fit in, how to help you, and not hinder. One dad told me that he felt left out because he couldn't feed the baby. And when he came home from work, the baby was often sleeping. Also, it is important to consider the changes in your sexual relationship with the birth of your baby. Your spouse/

partner may feel neglected or feel that your relationship is being neglected because of the increased focus on the baby. In addition to the changes in your body, you, mama, are so tired. Although I am not saying that it is our responsibility as new moms to care for our spouses while caring for a newborn, it's important for both partners to acknowledge how the parent who did not give birth may feel about this change in family dynamics. Both of you need to share your feelings regarding all these changes, which, at times, can be overwhelming.

## Communication With Your Partner

Communication with your spouse/partner is essential. Whether it is sending text messages during the day or carving out 15 minutes for adult conversation while the baby sleeps, tell your partner that this is important to you for your relationship. When you feel comfortable, hire a babysitter and go out for that date night. Someone told me this 19 years ago and I will never forget it: "It is important to stay connected with your husband. You don't want to look at each other 18 years later once your kid goes to college and have nothing to say to each other."

Whether this is your first baby or your third baby, eventually they will grow up. While you will always be a mother, it is important to maintain your relationship with your partner because that is the foundation on which your children are being raised. I hope my husband and I are setting a good example for our 3 teenagers that, yes, it is important to care for yourself and nurture the relationship, our marriage.

While writing this chapter and seeing patients in my clinic, I walked into an examination room. I greeted the parents, who were there with their 1-month old baby. The mom instantly began to cry. After a little visit, it became apparent that mom had wanted a baby for so long; she had a career and had been married for quite a while. And though she was understandably exhausted, she felt guilty for wanting some time off, some time away from the baby. Her husband, a really hands-on dad, told me that he is just trying to follow her lead, taking and feeding the baby when he gets home. I then asked them, "When are you going out, just the 2 of you?" Her face lit up. She looked at her husband and said that when his mother comes to see the baby the following week, they could go out on a date while grandma watches the baby.

I understand that everyone's situation is different. You may not have family or friends close by. You may not trust someone with your baby. I totally get that. But whether you go out to a restaurant, order take-out food and watch a movie, or sit on your porch with a glass of wine, it is important to carve out some alone time with your spouse/partner. If you have older children, set an appropriate bedtime for them so you and your partner can have some time alone. Talk with neighbors and friends who also have young children and get references for a reliable babysitter. This may mean that you bathe, feed, and put your baby down in the crib before you leave for date night. You do what makes you feel comfortable and safe.

## INTIMACY WITH YOUR PARTNER

Many aspects of the relationship with your spouse/partner are affected by the birth of your baby. Intimacy is an important aspect to consider, but it is often not discussed between couples. Remember, the physical changes along with your emotional and hormonal changes during this early postpartum period can affect your desire for intimacy. For many mothers, feeling unattractive while also being tired and even being isolated directly impact your overall feelings. Mom may feel disconnected from others, especially if there is limited interaction as a result of staying home to care for the baby. For many mothers, not being able to interact with other adults, whether socially or within a work environment, can make them feel even more isolated. This may cause resentment toward the spouse who continues to leave the house and interacts with others at work. It is normal for moms to feel out of sync with the outside world, and this has become increasingly the norm for mothers who gave birth during the COVID pandemic. Leaving the house or having visitors is a valid fear for new moms who are protecting their babies and themselves from the SARS-CoV-2 virus.

I remember after my husband came home from work, after having my second baby, I immediately asked him about his work day. I wanted specifics about the patients he saw, their aliments, and what he did to help them. I remember feeling a bit annoyed that he didn't really want to talk about work (understandably) while cuddling our son and playing with our toddler daughter. But for me, hearing about his work was a reprieve. I missed work and adult interaction since I was at home 10 hours a day with 2 children in diapers.

It is important to remember that the father/nonbirthing parent is also going through emotional changes during this period. Although they aren't facing the physicality of the postpartum period, your spouse/partner may feel neglected as your attention is focused on the baby. Your spouse may also be nervous about getting too close to you physically. Whether it is pain from the delivery, a healing c-section scar, or painful breasts from nursing, your spouse/partner may not want to touch you for fear of causing you further discomfort. It is also important to realize that certain aspects of intimacy are not recommended in those first 6 weeks after delivery.

But I want to remind you that it is so important to communicate with your spouse/partner about how you are feeling, both physically and emotionally. Acknowledge all of the changes you are feeling, and talk about it opening. Also, encourage your partner to talk about their feelings as well. Remember, this postpartum period will not last forever. Communication, understanding, and even a healthy dose of laughter will help both of you get through all these changes.

## CULTURAL SCENARIOS

Many moms reading this may be thinking, yeah, right, I can't leave my baby to enjoy myself. That's ridiculous. In many cultures, including my Indian culture, leaving your baby or child to go out on an adult-only date was unheard of when my kids were younger. Sadly, there tended to be a great deal of judgment—the assumption, the expectation that we, as mothers, are always supposed to be "on." Caring for our babies, our children.

Our needs come last. The marriage is not a priority while having babies and raising children.

Soon after my third child was born, we were invited to a large Indian gathering. After thanking my friend on the phone, I asked if I should get a babysitter or bring the kids. Her response: "Of course, the whole family should come. You are the only one who ever gets a babysitter!" Although I was taken aback, I didn't care about the criticism. I guess by the third child, I was used to unnecessary judgmental comments. Starting with our first child, my husband and I had established the importance of making time for each other. And between juggling kids and call schedules over the years, how we make time for each other and what we do looks different and will continue to change. You need to do whatever works for you, your spouse, and your growing family.

## So What Is Considered a Drink?

And as discussed in Chapter 7, for my breastfeeding mothers, you can have that cocktail or 1 glass of wine and not have to "pump and dump." If you know you'll be out for more than 3 hours, it is a good idea to pump before leaving the house so you are not engorged, uncomfortable, or leaking while you are out. Yes, that can happen, so plan accordingly.

So just imagine you have that special alone time, whether it's 1 hour or 3, no baby with you, no diaper bag, no children. You sit down at the table and take a deep breath. I want you to relax. After the waiter takes your drink order, what do you and your husband/partner do next?

Dietary Guidelines:

One drink

12 ounces of 5% beer

8 ounces of 7% malt liquor

5 ounces of 12% wine

0.5 ounce of 40% (80 proof) liquor

## JUST THE TWO OF US ALONE

While mamas are exhausted and need some time alone during this postpartum period, some fathers are actually quite hesitant about leaving the baby for a date night. Again, I cannot over-emphasize the importance of communication. Please talk with your spouse about how important it is to have some adult time alone. Reiterate the fact that this is good for you and your mental health, which, in turn, is good for the baby.

Although it may be upsetting that your partner just doesn't understand, having this discussion is important. Frequently, once spouses return to work, they are immersed in their regular schedule, having adult conversations and getting out of the house. The parent who is not at home all day with a newborn has *no* idea how hard it is. After a day of nursing, pumping, changing diapers, and doing laundry, I remember craving adult conversation once my husband came home. Again, not everyone feels this way, but when you have that need, that desire to spend time with your spouse, *tell* him or her. There is *no* guilt in feeling that you just want some time away with the person you are in a relationship with.

> ### My Special Message to All the New Dads and Partners Out There
>
> Hi dads and partners, please take your wife/partner out for date night. She deserves it. Signed, your friendly board-certified pediatrician (and mom of 3). OK, you can give the book back to her now.
>
> Remember my mantra? *Happy and healthy mama equals happy and healthy baby.*

After having a baby, it is natural for things in your marriage to change. The relationship may feel different now—not bad, not good—just different. Sometimes, that is hard to accept. You sense that certain loss of freedom, of being able to go out and do what you used to do, and it's OK to feel sad about that. This does not mean you are a bad mom or doing something wrong. This is nothing to feel guilty about. You are growing your family, and this is just a different stage of your marriage/relationship; it is a change for you as a mom as well as for your partner.

Once your babies grow up, they will eventually leave the house and establish their own lives. When that happens, it may be just you and your spouse. So don't put your marriage on the back burner while having babies and raising children. Although your babies and children will take priority many, if not most, times, it is important for you and your spouse/partner to nurture your relationship so it continues to grow and strengthen through good times and bad.

After your last child leaves the house, when you look at your spouse, you don't want to be looking at a stranger, right?

## BOTH PARTNERS ARE WORKING

When you get home from work, mom has been working all day too. Even though there may be bottles in the sink and the laundry is not done, a new baby is a full-time job, and sometimes her day has been more tiring than yours. It is important to remember that maternity leave is *not* a vacation or time off. Far from it. Mom is healing and trying to rest while caring for a brand new baby.

To all the spouses/partners reading this, whether this is the first, second, or third baby, each household and each situation is different. And just as you are adjusting to the new changes, mama may not know what she truly needs at that particular time. You know your wife/partner well. As the parent who did not give birth, you need to anticipate some of her needs. And if you don't know or aren't sure, just ask. Remember, communication is key.

## What Can Your Partner Do for You, Mama?

Talk to your partner and explain what they can do to help you through this postpartum period. Prepare a list and describe what is most helpful to you. Here are some suggestions:

- Get up at night to feed, change, and burp the baby. Go to another room so mom can get a restful sleep.
- Offer to take the baby for a walk to give mama time to herself.
- Dive in and start doing chores: laundry, dishes, cooking, or cleaning the bottles.
- Care for the newborn so mama can have quality time with the older child(ren).
- Help the older kids with their tasks, chores, and homework.
- Bring home mom's favorite takeout for dinner.
- Bring her a glass of water while she is breastfeeding.
- Make her breakfast before you leave for work and/or dinner once you get home.
- Book a massage for mama or send her for a pedicure/manicure, while you arrange for a babysitter.
- When mom is out, do *not* call or text her when you feel over-whelmed with a crying newborn or cranky toddler.
- Nudge mom to go out with friends or work out even if she is hesitant.
- Keep the kids busy so mom can take a nice long shower or bath without interruption.
- When in doubt, ask, "How can I be helpful to you?"

Helping your partner with these responsibilities can go a long way during this very stressful time.

CHAPTER 13

# Role of Social Media

SOCIAL MEDIA/noun /sōSHəl ˈmēdēə/: websites and applications that enable users to create and share content or to participate in social networking

A new mom came into my office for her baby's 1-month checkup. She had had a really difficult time getting pregnant. She and her husband wanted a baby for so long and had many doctor appointments. She was ecstatic when she found out she was pregnant. She chronicled much of her pregnancy on social media for others to read. Her outfits, the lighting, her pregnancy journey, and countdown to motherhood were all beautiful to see and read about. I walked into the examination room to find her sobbing. I handed her a few tissues and she began to share. She felt like she wasn't good enough. Breastfeeding was difficult, her baby cried all the time, and she was sleep-deprived. She hadn't told anyone but felt that her relationship with her husband had changed. I asked her if she had talked with some of her new-mom friends as a form of support. Do you know what she told me? She looked right at me and said, "No, because I see them on social media and they are doing everything right."

## HOW WE USE SOCIAL MEDIA CAN AFFECT US DIFFERENTLY

While there are many outlets for peer support on the internet and social media, much of the information is based on opinion and posted by people who are not experts.

> 66
>
> Do not compare your reality to someone else's highlight reel.
>
> 99

I remember hearing this phrase years ago when my daughter received a cell phone and was on social media. (Navigating the teenage years is an entirely different book!) I was trying to teach her how to navigate social media, and what I saw, not only as a mother, but as a physician and woman, truly alarmed me. Women of all ages, many who were mothers, were feeling inadequate based on the images they were viewing on social media. When I was in the early stages of motherhood, I only had to contend with the images I saw on television or on the magazine covers in the grocery check-out aisle. Headlines like "bounce back to your prepregnancy body in 6 weeks!" or photos of skinny-looking celebrity women with perfect makeup taking their kids to the park (never mind the entourage of people helping them in the wings). With technology at our fingertips and every social media app accessible at all times, the onslaught of images and posts is never-ending. I observed this not only as a mother but as a physician who sees pregnant and postpartum women in my office every day. I also experienced this with friends and neighbors who were new mothers.

Studies show that exposure to social media can increase anxiety and/or depression. In fact, it can directly impact your mental health and emotional wellness. It can also affect your sleep.

So when you combine sleep deprivation with postpartum hormones, it is not surprising that social media can make women feel worse, a lot worse. New mothers are already struggling with so many unknowns. Some will question if they are doing the right thing and others will feel weighed down by what seem like life-altering decisions.

I can assure you, however, that whether you decide to formula feed or breastfeed, whether you go back to work or stay at home, and whether you had a natural birth or cesarean delivery, your baby will be fine. I often see moms sacrifice their own physical health and mental well-being because they think that is what they are *supposed* to do for their baby.

## SOCIAL MEDIA CAN OBSCURE OUR REALITY

Social media often obscures reality. It can make many of us feel inadequate, guilty, and as if we're not being good mothers. Comparison is the thief of joy.

It is always difficult to match expectation with reality. Whether it's the Pinterest mom or the woman who is back in her pre-pregnancy jeans within a month, all the images affect us, even if we think we are just scrolling. A psychologist I work with told me that the images we see, what we bombard ourselves with, all affect our brain, even if we think we are not actively engaged.

A friend and I were talking about how things have changed since we had our kids almost 20 years ago. We had to contend with the magazine covers showing celebrities looking like the perfect moms, having it all together, and wearing the perfect outfit. I still detest those magazines that scream we have to be a certain size or weight by a certain time in the postpartum period. Mamas, you are contending with a lot, so much more than I had to 15 to 20 years ago. And although you may realize that what you are seeing and reading isn't always accurate, it can and will affect you.

One of my mothers brought her baby to my office for a 1-month well-child (health supervision) visit. I noticed a definite change in her mood. After examining the baby, I sat down and started to delve into what may have been bothering her. She began to cry and said that she had been searching online, which was not only overwhelming but was also making her feel as if she was doing everything wrong.

## Dangers of Dr Google

Many of you will point out that you get a lot of support from various Facebook groups. Yes, that's true. Finding peer support on social media has been a positive experience for many new moms. However, when searching for medical advice online, especially during such a vulnerable time, the results can be misleading and even dangerous. Whether it's information about breastfeeding, infant development, immunizations, postpartum weight loss, or even maternal mental health, heeding advice based on opinion is worrisome.

This is a prime example of the dangers of Dr Google. Infants are undergoing an often unnecessary procedure based on what stressed-out and sleep-deprived mothers are finding online. Just imagine that your baby is crying or you are struggling with

> " I read online about the risks of tongue-tie [ankyloglossia] and not getting it taken care of since that will put my baby at risk for future speech delay. He was breastfeeding fine, but I had other family members who had issues with it and speech. And now after the procedure, I feel so bad, he is in so much pain. "

breastfeeding, it's 3 am, and you are *exhausted*. You start googling or searching online based on what you're experiencing. No doubt you will find hundreds of answers. However, as I said in the introduction, my goal is to provide evidence-based information along with real-life advice. You can almost always find something online to verify what you think or what others have told you. But much of what is written and/or posted is faulty advice that is made to look like fact. It isn't. Trust me, most people giving medical advice online have not spent hours reading and analyzing scientific articles, which is necessary when making medical recommendations.

While the value of online peer support cannot be underestimated, please keep that separate from online medical advice that can adversely affect your baby and you.

Of course, I am always willing to listen to parental concerns, but I ask parents what they have heard and/or read. This gives me insight into their beliefs and fears. When I go through the evidence based on the points they have raised, I do so from the point of view of a pediatrician and a mother. Validating mamas' feelings is important. And I get it, I totally get it. While social media may not have been around when my kids were born, I listened to so much unsolicited advice from other women and mothers of all ages. Looking back, I realize that although something may have worked for them, that did not mean it was going to work for my baby, my family, or me. Also, I think it is reasonable to question someone's motivation for saying and/or writing these things. What may appear to be supportive may actually be harmful.

Although many mamas appreciate the evidence I provide in the office, that doesn't mean they will take my advice. And that is OK. My goal is to give information, whether it is via my online presence or this book, so *you* can make an informed decision. One that is right for you and your baby.

*Remember, I went to school a lot longer than Dr Google.* My moms always chuckle when I say that.

To all my mamas, please use social media and online sites only if they help you. If they stress you out or make you feel less than—like you are a bad mother or everyone else is doing things right—then please take a break.

### Sometimes You Need to Unplug

Practically, you can set a time limit on your apps. You can have your smartphone shut everything down (except necessary functions such as phone, text, video chat, maps) after a designated time. I don't care how old you are, or how many years you have been a mother, *all* of us can benefit from this downtime. Please don't fall into the trap of comparing yourself to others, as you have no idea what their true story is and are only seeing what they choose to share. As I said earlier, social media can have adverse effects on your mental health.

I encourage you to use online peer support if you find it helpful. However, if it causes you stress or worry or makes you question yourself, then that is not the right space for you. During the COVID-19 pandemic, much of the individual, group, and peer support moved online. Again, these virtual outlets should be helping you and making you feel better and stronger. Not diminishing you.

Finally, please be wary of falling down the rabbit hole of searching for medical advice online. While there are physicians who have a valid online presence, you need to know from whom you are getting advice. Please consider their medical education and background, as well as question what their motivation may be by posting certain things. Again, I hope this book will serve as a resource, not only to help guide you on all things fourth trimester, but also to empower you to advocate for yourself and your baby.

Bear in mind, having an opinion about what it means to be a mother is much easier than actually doing it, every single day. You got this, mama. And remember, you have me along for the journey.

Again, what's my mantra? *Happy and healthy mama (this includes mental health) equals happy and healthy baby.*

# CHAPTER 14

# Mommy Guilt: It's Real Folks

> **GUILT**/noun/gilt/: the fact of having committed a specified or implied offense or crime
>
> verb: to make (someone) feel guilty, especially in order to induce them to do something

Early on in my first pregnancy, when my baby was the size of a grape, a distant family member who had decided to stay at home with her own children said loudly to me in a busy restaurant, "Good moms don't work." It was 2001, and I still remember that comment like it was yesterday. I was shocked, I was embarrassed, and I was angry. Regardless of whether she deserved an explanation, I felt a great need to explain myself to her. I felt like I had to defend my choice to work. I was already feeling insecure and scared, and, sadly, this woman only worsened those feelings.

This scenario happened to me again. I was at my neighborhood holiday block party, but this time I had my 2 youngest kids, still in diapers, in tow. I was alone as my husband was working most weekends. I was completely and utterly sleep-deprived. A neighbor who found out that I was a pediatrician said to me, "I don't know how you leave your own children to go take care of other peoples' kids." To provide some context, this woman had decided to stay at home with her kids when they were born, but she also hired a nanny to watch them 6 days a week.

Another really good friend and fellow physician who sets up health care programs in Central America was attending her son's school concert. Because of the nature of her career and busy travel schedule, her husband—the father of their 3 kids—decided to put his career on hold to be a stay-at-home father. A decision they made together. Prior to the start of the performance, the principal was making announcements and welcoming the parents and families. He made a point of saying, "Oh, it's nice to see Mrs. Jones here today."

## MOMMY GUILT IS EVERYWHERE

I am sharing these stories with you not to disparage anyone's choices to stay at home with their kids or go back to work, but I want to highlight the reality that these statements not only impact how we feel about ourselves as mothers but intensify and often worsen our mommy guilt.

What I want to convey is that mommy guilt will come at you from all directions: friends, families, other women, neighbors, social media, and even colleagues in the workplace. People will comment on your decision to bottle feed or breastfeed. You will definitely hear comments about your choice to stay home to care for your baby versus returning to a career outside the home. The stories I could share with you would fill a few more chapters. Over the past 20 years, I have witnessed less judgment and more acceptance of the choices we make as mothers, but guilt, judgment, and unsolicited advice continue. Based on my own experiences, what I see in my practice, and how I counsel new mothers, I hope to help you acknowledge it, manage it, and let it go. What I have learned is that if it doesn't serve you as a mother and if it doesn't add positivity to you, your family, or your children, then it doesn't deserve your time, attention, or energy.

### Acknowledge It

Over the past 20 years, and 3 kids, 2 states, and 5 houses later, I can tell you this: Change is good. I have done it all. I have been the stay-at-home mom, putting my career on hold while volunteering with the PTA. I have also worked as a physician and researcher full-time, spending my time in the office, seeing patients, and having some really long commutes. I have worked night shifts caring for babies and children in a pediatric emergency department. And you may be surprised to know that all of my kids were younger than 5 through these changes.

When I moved to a new state, I started to work part-time as a physician and part-time at home as a mother. Whether it's 40/60, 50/50, or 75/25, my work-life balance continues to change. What I am saying is that depending on your circumstances, where you live, the ages of your children, and your career goals, you (along with your spouse/partner) and only you know what will work for you, your child(ren), your partner, your family. What works for your family this year may be different in 1 year, 3 years, or 5 years. Use the options available to you—whether that is flexible work hours, the ability to work remotely, or flexibility regarding household finances—to your advantage to help you decide what serves you and your family best at that time. Keep in mind, your decision is not set in stone; you can and probably will change as time goes on.

What I am trying to say is that during my numerous postpartum journeys, I discovered that change was good for my family, my children, and me. There was judgment from others, as well as self-criticism. Though the changes we make during our postpartum journey may leave us feeling uncomfortable and unsettled, just know that you are doing what works best for your family, your baby, and you.

### Manage It

My husband and I had to make decisions based on what worked for our family and our careers. What worked for us at various times during the past 20 years included having a nanny versus taking our children to a child care center because of our unpredictable schedules. To gain more control over my schedule, I took a job that allowed me to do shift work as a pediatrician in an emergency center. This then morphed into my husband working all-night shifts so he was home during the day while I resurrected my career as a professor and researcher, which required more travel. Whatever you decide today, tomorrow, or even next month will change down the road. And that is OK, I promise. Your baby and any older children will not only be fine with these changes, they will thrive! You are teaching them resilience and showing them that change is good. Your actions are setting an amazing example for them. I know as mamas we want to have control over as many things as possible, but you don't need to plan everything right now. Because no matter how much you try to plan, babies, children, and especially teenagers find joy in completely upending those plans.

### Learn to Let It Go

Another aspect of mommy guilt? Yes, you guessed it. Taking time for ourselves. Away from our baby. Away from the children. Away from the house. Doing something for ourselves that gives us joy, makes us feel less stressed, and re-energizes us. Raise your hand if this is you. Time and time again, I see this with so many moms, especially new moms. Mothers often find it difficult to give themselves permission to take time out for themselves. We tend to focus on the newborn, older children, our partners, the house, cooking, cleaning, and organizing. You and your needs are often last on your to-do list. However, health is not simply physical health, it is also taking care of your mental health.

While you acknowledge your feelings of guilt and may even be affected by the judgment of others, I hope that, with time and support, you can put into perspective what is important and what works best for you and your family. And as you move forward and do what is right for you and aligns best with your family's needs and values, please let go of all that judgment and self-criticism.

## SPECIFIC STRATEGIES TO MANAGE YOUR MOMMY GUILT

I want to provide you with specific strategies that will allow you to manage your mommy guilt, improve your mental health, and minimize the stress you may be feeling. No matter the age of your newborn and any other child(ren), you can and should be taking time for yourself.

### A Simple 4%

A few years ago, as I was preparing a lecture for young female physicians about work-life balance, I found a statistic. It was 4%. Four percent seems pretty miniscule, right? Well guess what? When translated into a day, a full 24 hours, 4% is 1 hour. So mama, listen to me when I say this. Taking 1 hour a day for yourself is not huge; it's actually the opposite. Four percent of your day is a small part of the day. Whether you have to negotiate this hour with your partner, your child care facility, your job outside the home, or your other tasks, I want you to take an hour for yourself every day. OK, I know my new mamas reading this are thinking that I have 3 heads and they may want to throw the book at me. But hear me out. I often tell my new mamas to start with 30 minutes a day or even every other day. Whatever works. And yes, I tell their partners, husbands, or grandmothers sitting beside them because they play an important role in making this happen. Your partner or other people in your life may not know that this is what you need. Again, no one can read your mind. If they aren't hearing this from a physician or someone else, then you must tell them. Even if you feel bad about asking or unsettled about leaving the baby, you will appreciate that time to yourself. As a mother, you are a natural caregiver. You take care of everyone else and everything else. Remember the safety announcement we always hear before the airplane takes off? Put on your own oxygen mask before helping others? Well, I am here to tell you that it is OK to take care of you. Doctor's orders!

### Dedicate Time for Yourself

Whether it is sleeping, going for a walk (without having to worry about a stroller or diaper bag), working out, or meeting a friend for coffee or even a drink, please do this for yourself. It will recharge you. It will refresh you. It will re-energize you as a mother. I realize, especially in those early weeks and months, that the thought of leaving your newborn can be too much. But your baby will be fine. Your baby is safe. Your baby won't be scarred for life. In fact, your baby will feed off your relaxed mood and happiness. Your mental health and well-being directly impact and benefit your baby. Remember my mantra: *Happy and healthy mama equals happy and healthy baby.*

### Learn to Say No

One thing I have learned as a mother and a physician is that women need to learn to be comfortable saying *no*. You don't have to be rude. And you don't need to feel bad or guilty when you say no. I want you to learn this very important word. Repeat after me. No! This is a gigantic step in setting boundaries in so many aspects of your life. Whether it's saying no to people coming over in the early days to visit your newborn, or turning down a work trip that will keep you away from your baby, or even saying no to volunteering at your toddler's preschool, learning to say no is important. As mothers, we are often overstretched and over-committed. Remember, you are not saying no just for the sake of saying no but to stand up for what is best for you, your baby, and your family. Setting boundaries now will not only help you as a mom, but also as a woman, which, in turn, will help your family.

As women and as mothers, we tend to take on so many things, and continue to add tasks and responsibilities, whether it is caring for the newborn, caring for our spouse and older children, or even doing household tasks. Again, as mothers we continue to add. But we often do this without subtracting. We rarely take things off our plates, and, as a result, we often put ourselves last.

Instead, by taking things off our plates, we can prioritize our needs to best take care of ourselves and our families.

Over the years, as my family has grown, I have learned to ask myself the following questions:

- Personal requests: Some examples are chairing the PTA fund-raiser, hosting Thanksgiving dinner, or attending mommy and me newborn classes. Ask yourself: Is this fun? Does this bring me joy? Does this allow me to spend quality time with my children, my family?

- Career-oriented requests: Before you commit to another board or committee roster, give a professional lecture, or lead a project, ask yourself: Is this lucrative? Will this further my career? Is this worth the time away from my family?

I believe these questions will help you form a framework before saying yes. As your family grows, so do your responsibilities. Don't feel forced to say yes because you fear you would be letting someone down if you said no.

When my third child was born, my female neighbors were so excited that we had now become a family of 5. When we came home from the hospital, they were all there to welcome us. One of my closest friends, whose children were older, gave me the best advice. She said, "In that postpartum period, in those early days, we are in the *physical exhaustion* phase, whereas when our babies get older, especially those teen years, we are in the *mental exhaustion* phase." Our responsibilities as mothers, what we worry about, and our children's needs continually change. However, it doesn't matter how old they are. We are and always will be mothers.

Aside from the physical tasks of feeding/nursing, changing diapers, and waking up at all hours of the night, the mental load we mamas carry is *huge*. The mental load, also known as cognitive labor, refers to the invisible load mothers carry in managing the household and family. It's not about doing the actual task, but overseeing the task and making sure the task is completed. Think of those endless to-do lists running in your head that, at least for me, may even keep you up at night. Mama, you don't need to be a martyr. You need to rest, recover, and rejuvenate during this postpartum period. Moreover, the standards and boundaries you set now will be important in the years to follow. Although you can plan for some of this during pregnancy (see Chapter 4), developing strategies for beyond the postpartum period is essential, not only to maintain your sanity but also to have some time for yourself.

## DIVISION OF LABOR

First and foremost, as a new mother you need to learn how to delegate. You cannot be the sole parent who cooks, cleans, cares for the new baby, pays the bills, takes care of the house and yardwork, and cares for any older siblings. The household duties can be delegated and completed by others; you cannot and must not do them alone. What does this mean? It is important for your spouse/partner to be involved, and together you need to create a plan for these various child care and household duties. Aside from nursing, your significant other can be involved in the care of the newborn (refer to Chapter 5). For parents with older children, even toddlers, they too can help out around the house. Whether it's picking up their toys or, for older children, putting their dishes into the dishwasher, you are setting the standard, the expectations for all family members, even the youngest ones. You can even initiate these tasks before the new baby arrives. Remember, mama, you are not the maid or a short order cook (yes, I've used this line in my house).

Let me give you a piece of advice (you'll thank me later). When your partner takes over various duties and tasks, realize that he or she *will* do things differently from you. And that is OK. Just accept that. What matters is that things get done while tasks are taken off your list. So you can rest and take time for yourself.

Many of us mamas do things a certain way within a certain time frame, but when we delegate, things will be done differently and under different circumstances and timing. Although it may be difficult for you to accept initially, letting go will pay off because your partner will be taking responsibility for various tasks so you don't have to. In addition to decreasing your mental load, it will also empower your spouse/partner, who often feels helpless in those early days after bringing a newborn home. Voicing what you need and asking for help are important. Tell your partner what you need and ask your friends and family for assistance. As I said earlier, communication is key.

## WORK-LIFE BALANCE

Regardless of whether you are a stay-at-home mom or work outside of the home, 99.9% of the time, society designates mom as the default parent. Why? This is most likely based on years of antiquated gender roles based on societal norms. Time and time again, whether among friends and family or even in my pediatric practice, the mother is expected to care for the newborn and manage all things pertaining to child care. However, your spouse/partner is not there to help you; as a parent, this person is (or should be) an equal partner when it comes to child-rearing, as well as all other household and familial duties.

I give lectures on the topic of work-life balance, which is defined as how people spend and manage their time outside of work. Whether you work at home or outside the home, the work aspect often bleeds into the life aspect. This is especially true for mothers. During these lectures, I sometimes hear this comment:

While that may be true for more families these days, the traditional societal expectation has been that mothers are the default parent, whether or not they work full-time. In many cases, moms are still the ones responsible for taking the kids to their doctors'

> " My partner is the stay-at-home dad, while I work full-time. He does the bulk of the child care and household management "

appointments, joining baby play groups to give the child the socialization needed, picking up kids from school, getting them to after-school activities, or attending the concert and recitals. Regardless of the internal family structure, the assumption often is that mom will be the first one to tend to her child's needs.

When my second child was a baby and my oldest was a toddler, I was on maternity leave and had the opportunity to travel to a medical conference. I cannot tell you how many friends and neighbors called and offered my husband help while I was away (for just 3 days!). One person said to him, "It's so great how you babysit your kids." What? Although, thankfully, that sentiment is starting to change, society places certain expectations on mothers as *the* primary caregiver for our babies, children, and families. These expectations can and often do worsen our mommy guilt. Although changes are taking place, I continue to see such expectations placed on younger women and mothers I work with, whether it is from family, friends, child care settings, or even the workplace.

When there is judgment or there are certain expectations you feel you need to meet (which there will be) or you have mommy guilt (which you will feel), I want you to stop beating yourself up. Forgive yourself. And give yourself grace. Did you hear me? Grace! You are *one* person, and let me tell you, mama, you are doing the best you can. Yes, you will forget. Yes, you will mess up. It's called being human. And every single mother reading this needs to support other mothers. Please support each other! It means so much to hear from women who are or have been where we are, especially during the postpartum stage. I would have loved knowing that I was not alone in my feelings.

Mama, you do not need to do it all alone. We are all doing the best we can with the resources we have. And, yes, sometimes we need more resources. So when you do, please remember to reach out and ask for help, whether it is from other mothers, friends, family members, your spouse/partner, or doctor. And you are definitely not the only one feeling this way.

I was shopping one day when I saw a mom juggling 3 kids, 2 in the cart and a baby wrapped on her chest. Not surprisingly, one of the toddlers was having a meltdown because he wanted something in the check-out line. The look of frustration on her face was so familiar. I remember being in similar situations and shaming myself for not even being able to get grocieries, feeling that I was doing everything wrong. I approached her and said, "Honestly, just tell the manager to keep your cart aside so you can come back for it later. It's OK for you to come back later, you're juggling a lot." I don't know what she ended up doing as I quickly walked away after she thanked me. However, I think receiving that validation from other mothers about how unglamorous and difficult it is to be a mama would help so many of us who have been, and continue to be, in challenging parenting situations. We'll feel less alone when we realize there is a large community of mothers, just like you, just like me, who have been there and understand exactly what you are feeling.

## GOING BACK TO WORK ADVICE

> We expect women to work like they don't have children and raise children as if they don't work. ~Unknown

For my mamas who are planning to return to work or are already working outside the home, it is challenging. As working moms, you will always feel like you are doing 2 or more jobs. The costs of motherhood are real. Many mothers feel conflicted about returning to the workplace, and study after study shows that work policies do not favor women. In fact, the United States is in last place for its lack of support for working mothers. Lack of paid maternity leave and inflexible work hours do not make things easier for us mamas. What happens when your child has a fever and is unable to go to child care or your nanny becomes ill? Mom often ends up needing to stay home with the baby. This can and likely will affect your work colleagues.

Deciding which parent will stay home is based on various factors, such as work responsibilities, flexibility, and financial constraints. In many cases, because of traditional family roles (along with the fact that women are often paid less than men), the mother often is the one who decides to stay home with the new baby. But because this is not always a given, it is important to have this discussion with your spouse/partner based on your family circumstances and desires.

Twenty years later, young mothers still tell me that the preschool has scheduled the school activity or Mother's Day tea at 11 in the morning! I highly doubt that many of us can just drop everything to attend an activity in the middle of the morning. To be honest, it infuriates me that this still occurs. What may help, if you are in this situation or will be in the future, is to ask your child's teacher to be considerate of your work schedule and the importance of getting certain dates in advance so you can plan accordingly. Still, if you work outside the home, you may miss certain school activities and events. I know it's hard, and you feel sad and guilty. But your child will be fine. Maybe your spouse/partner, a relative, or even a good friend can attend the event. As working moms, we often have to pick and choose, but just know that there are many ways to ensure that your child feels loved.

Work-life balance is hard, it really is. And the lack of supportive policies for working moms is having long-term effects. While writing this book, I read a column that stated that college-educated women underestimate the demands of motherhood and the difficulties of combining working and parenting. This adds to our mental load and overall stress. Moms working outside the home often feel that they should be able to do it all, both at home and at work.

While this may not change anytime soon, it is important for you to know, mama, that you can stop trying to reach these ideals at home and work. What you are doing now, right now, caring for your baby, your family, and yourself, makes you Superwoman. However, there are no awards for working to the point of mental exhaustion. There are no awards for how little sleep you get. There are no awards for how much you volunteer at your toddler's preschool. There are no awards for the number of months or years you breastfeed. You need to find a schedule that works best for you. You need to find time to meet your own needs. Does that mean finding time to do something you love, such as reading a book, going to a movie with a friend, or working out? Although finding that balance may not always be easy, I am here to tell you that it can be done. You, mama, are worth it. So please, do this for *you*.

At an orchestra concert, a friend approached me and said, "Wow you're like Wonder Woman." I know she meant it as a compliment, but then I told her about how I forgot to sign my daughter's permission slip and she was the only kid in her class who wasn't allowed to attend the field trip. And you know what? My daughter was OK. Sure, she was disappointed, but she got over it. I felt terrible at first, but I apologized and then let it go. What's done is done, and in the big scheme of things, my child is OK. Our children are allowed to be disappointed, and, believe me, it's not the end of the world. I decided to forgive myself for messing up and gave myself grace. So though all of you mamas are Wonder Woman in my book, I do not want you drowning in stress to hold yourself to some unrealistic ideal.

You also need to be cautious and limit your social media intake. A considerable amount of evidence shows why social media makes moms feel so awful. Mom guilt comes in all sizes and situations and is very relatable. Mothers have told me that they don't know how these Pinterest moms do it. A mother of 3, who was one of my fitness instructors, told me, "I go on Facebook and just feel like I'm not doing it right." A friend, a single working mom, said, "I can't go on Facebook during the holidays. I can't decorate like that or afford all those gifts." And time and time again, I hear some rendition of "look how skinny she is!"

Putting down your smartphone and pausing your scrolling may be hard, but you need to stop comparing your reality to someone else's highlight reel.

Whether you are a new postpartum mother, or a mother of 3, your needs as a mother and as a woman will change, just as your child grows and their development changes. Find other like-minded women, other mothers who are in your life space. While many of you have forever friends in your life, it is important to find your tribe. These mothers will be instrumental as you navigate whatever stage of motherhood you are in. Whether it is those early postpartum months, the preschool phase, or those teen (!) years, things rarely go as planned regardless of how much you prepare. With that in mind, leaning on other moms for support and advice while you relax and unwind is not only fun but essential for your mental health.

Whatever you do, mama, remember that love is the key ingredient. It is not about the quantity of time but the quality of the time spent with your children. It is about the moments that your child(ren) will remember, not the stuff, the things. As a mother who used to worry incessantly about the small things and carried an enormous amount of mommy guilt, especially as I returned to work, I learned that it does not matter if your baby received formula. It does not matter which sippy cup your baby used. It does not matter if you didn't take your infant to a mommy and me class or register for the *right* preschool. And it does not matter if you decided to stay at home or go back to work. Your baby is loved. And with that love your baby will grow and develop into a strong and happy child. Give yourself grace, mama, because you are doing a great job.

CHAPTER 15

# Maximizing Sleep as a New Mommy

## Really, It's Not a Myth!

> **SLEEP**/noun /slēp/: a condition of body and mind that typically recurs for several hours every night, in which the nervous system is relatively inactive, the eyes closed, the postural muscles relaxed, and consciousness practically suspended

Although advice you receive from friends and family and even from physicians will vary, my hope is that you will find something that works for you, your partner, your baby, and your family in this chapter. The goal is for you to find ways to maximize your sleep, mama.

> 66 I wish someone had told me that no matter how many pregnancy or baby books I read, nothing could've prepared me for the lack of sleep and how tired I would feel in those early weeks and months after coming home with my newborn. 99

You have just returned home with your newborn. You are excited to finally be back in your home. Everything is ready; the baby clothes are washed and put away, the monitor is plugged in, and the nursery is all decorated. Many new moms receive the advice to sleep when the baby sleeps, but what does that really mean? There are many books on the market about baby's sleep, but this chapter is different. Just like the rest of the book, the focus is on how you, as a mom, can maximize your sleep and rest with a new baby. No, I'm not delusional; it can happen. And that's what I'm here for—to help you find and navigate what works best for you, your baby, and your family. Again, one size does not fit all.

## YOUR BODY NEEDS SLEEP

Remember that you have just grown, nourished, and birthed a small human. Your body needs to rest and heal. Your body and your mind need sleep. Although some days and nights will be tougher than others, understand that as a new mother you can and will need to sleep. This rest is an essential part of your healing.

Most important, when baby sleeps, you need to sleep … or at least rest, mama. I know this sounds like a cliché, but there is some truth to it. After you are done feeding your baby, if someone is in the house to help you, please hand this person your infant and go straight to your room or another place in the house where you can lie down. I do not want you to start cooking, cleaning, or hopping on the computer to pay bills, and definitely do not start scrolling through your feed. During this time, you need to shut off your brain for a few hours and rest. For my mamas who are home alone throughout the day (this was me), after changing and swaddling the baby, put the baby into a safe space (crib, bassinette) for sleeping while you lie down in your own bed. Believe me, this is not always easy. As mothers, we have the urge to use this time to get other things done. Or you may be worrying about your baby and not be able to sleep. It may not happen right away, which is 100% normal, but you need to continue to try so it becomes a habit.

### Sleep Tips for Breastfeeding Mothers

As a pediatrician, I often am asked, "How can I sleep if I am nursing my baby every 2 hours?" This is a valid question. If you're nursing, it often seems (rightly so) that you are the only one who can feed your baby. As someone who breastfed, nursed, and pumped for all 3 children, I can attest to the fact that it is exhausting. And just because it is natural does *not* mean it's easy.

Those early weeks are extremely important (see Chapter 7) to establish your supply when breastfeeding. After those first few weeks, when your breast milk supply is well-established, I want you to start thinking about getting a longer stretch of sleep. Whether you have already started pumping breast milk or have formula available, this is the time you need to have a conversation with your spouse/partner or another family member who may be in your home.

While you are nursing your newborn every 1 to 2 hours, some babies may start to sleep for longer stretches of time around the 1-month mark. Again, every baby is different. Based on your baby's weight, development, and nutritional needs, your pediatrician will let you know how often and how much your baby should be feeding.

One common concern I hear is that if a nursing or pumping session is skipped at night, mom is covered in milk. This is true; your breasts will feel quite heavy, and often breast milk will have leaked onto your pajama top and even at times onto the bedsheets. Let's go back to an earlier example. When the baby wakes at 3 or 4 am, you will have quite a bit of breast milk. Go ahead and immediately nurse the baby. First, completely empty one breast before offering the second breast. If your baby doesn't take the second breast and/or you still feel full, get on your breast pump and completely empty those breasts. For my mamas who are exclusively pumping, then pump both breasts on waking and feed the fresh milk directly to the baby. Again, this will save you time from having to prepare a bottle of refrigerated breast milk.

As a mother, pediatrician, and breastfeeding medicine specialist, I am 100% in favor of breast milk for babies. However, my philosophy has always been that *some is better than none.* I don't want any mother to feel sad or guilty if her baby gets some formula. Of course, I know that is easier said than done. For various reasons, all of my children received formula, both in the early days and later months. But if you haven't started pumping or just don't want to, giving your baby 1 bottle of formula at night so you can sleep is OK. What good is it if you are walking around like a zombie, irritable, sleep-deprived, and not enjoying your baby? Mama, getting a solid 5 to 6 hours of sleep is important not only for your physical and mental health but also for your baby. If you do not want your baby to receive formula, then please start pumping once daily during the early morning hours (approximately 3 to 6 am) to start building up that supply so your partner can grab a bottle of breast milk for that feed in the middle of the night.

## Please Do Not Disturb a Sleeping Mom or Her Newborn

I suggest putting up a sign or note on your door so neighbors, friends, and delivery people do not ring the doorbell during the daytime, as it will only disturb you (and the baby) during the shorter rest periods. Also, for my fellow dog moms, it will prevent the dog from barking and waking up the baby and you. (Please find a sample doorbell sign on my website at NatashaMomMD.com.)

## Sleep Tips for Bottle-Feeding Mothers

For my mamas who are feeding the baby formula, if you decide to prepare the nighttime bottles ahead of time, that is fine. To save time for middle of the night feedings, you can put the powder formula in the bottle and just add the water at 3 am. But your partner is solely responsible for getting up with the baby, taking the baby to the kitchen, and preparing the formula bottle. I do not want you to be woken up to help.

## Sleep Tips When You Have Older Children

Many of my mamas with toddlers are wondering how they can rest when the newborn sleeps if they have a 2-year-old to entertain. In 2004, this was me. Getting your toddlers on a schedule is essential. However, even if they have been on a good schedule, expect them to regress, which is a normal developmental response to a new baby. During the day, when the baby is sleeping, bring your toddler into bed with you so she or he can flip through a book or watch an age-appropriate show or cartoon while you rest and sleep. My toddler learned to count and tell time from a famous fuzzy red puppet as I was trying to juggle her and her newborn brother. Depending on your toddler, I strongly encourage you to continue their regular nap time, and as the weeks ensue, try to coordinate that nap time with your newborn's sleep. Your toddler may not nap, and that's OK. But your toddler can learn to have *quiet time*. They can sit quietly in their crib or toddler bed with a book. Eventually, your toddler will lie down and even close their eyes for a bit. But even if your toddler doesn't fall asleep, you are establishing a quiet period that allows your toddler to rest while you and the baby are sleeping. Keep in mind that children, especially toddlers, thrive on a schedule and need adequate sleep, so don't be surprised if this scheduled quiet time allows your toddler to be well-rested and less irritable.

## HOW YOUR PARTNER CAN HELP

Whether you are a first-time mother or a seasoned mother, one thing I can tell you is that you can and will hear your baby at all times, including even the quietest peep. After her third child was born, a friend told me that I should sleep on my husband's side of the bed because he doesn't seem to hear the baby crying from over there. Hilarious, yet true. I literally had to shake my husband awake for him to get the baby out of the crib.

Whether it is your expressed breast milk or formula, you and your partner will need to navigate at least 1 of those feedings each night so you can get a longer stretch of sleep. For example, if you nurse the baby at 10 pm and the baby then sleeps until midnight or 1 am, your partner can then feed the baby with a bottle *while you sleep*. You are not to be woken up to get the bottle, mix the formula, or change the diaper. You *must* not be disturbed. Please make that clear to your partner. After that feed, the baby will most likely be hungry by 3 or 4 am, and that is when you wake up to nurse your baby. At this point, you have gotten approximately 5 to 6 hours of undisturbed sleep. I know it's shocking. When I see moms after a full stretch of sleep, I always say, "You feel like a new woman, don't you?" Sleep completely changes how you feel, not just at that moment but for the rest of the day. It improves your mood and allows you to enjoy the day so much more because you are well-rested.

As your baby grows, his or her sleep patterns will change based on nutritional and developmental needs. However, it is important to continue to negotiate the feeding schedule with your partner so you can get that 4- to 5-hour stretch of sleep.

Some of you may be thinking that because your spouse/partner works all day, they need their sleep so can't be expected to wake up and feed the baby. As I've explained in earlier chapters, the role of the mother often is based on cultural and societal expectations. As a result, the majority of the caregiving responsibilities will fall on you. But let's be clear. Just because you aren't leaving the house to go to work does *not* mean you are not working. Maternity leave is not a vacation or time off. It is work.

Your baby is lovely and precious but staying home all day with a newborn can be exhausting. Honestly, sometimes going to work with other adults gave me a break. Please do not let anyone tell you that what you are doing as a new mother is easier than going to work. It most definitely is not. Yes, your partner works hard but so do you. And that means that your partner's sleep is no more important than your sleep. I know it's hard, but you need to let go of that mommy guilt. Mama, you are not to be the sole caregiver for your baby. Your spouse/partner can feed and care for the baby so you can rest.

Although you may experience difficulty sleeping when you are home alone with the newborn, this should not be the case when an adult is at home with you. When your partner comes home from work and you need to sleep, please nurse or feed the baby and then give the baby to your partner. You also should ask your partner to take the newborn (and toddler) out of the house so you can sleep. Watching the baby in another room while you try to sleep does not count because you may have difficulty tuning out the cries and coos of the baby. When they leave the house, those sounds are not there to distract or worry you. As I said in Chapter 5, partners are not babysitters; they are capable of caring for and feeding the newborn—and you have to be OK with them doing it differently from the way you would do it.

I also want you to take a look at that postpartum plan you made during your pregnancy. Reach out to a family member, friend, or neighbor to come over. Perhaps that person can feed and hold the newborn while you take a shower and get some rest. Or ask them to take your toddler to the park so you can rest while your newborn sleeps. For many women (including me), asking for help is difficult. But please reach out and ask. Again, those couple of hours of rest will be so beneficial for your physical and mental health.

I can laugh about this memory now as my kids are older, but 16 years ago it was not funny. My husband had just arrived home. I remember it was a Sunday. I had been home all weekend with 2 kids under the age of 2 who were both in diapers. While I was happy to see my husband, I desperately needed sleep. My husband took both of the kids into the backyard to play. I hadn't even put my head down on the pillow when my toddler came running into my bedroom screaming that daddy dropped the baby! I sprinted out of bed and ran into the backyard. While the baby was fine, he was crying in my husband's arms. I took the baby and held him to calm him down. After the crying stopped, my husband explained that while he was outside with both kids, the baby crawled away from my husband to get to his sister who was on the swing. Needless to say, my husband got an earful of my anger and frustration. Of course, both kids were fine, and my husband realized how closely he needed to watch 2 kids. But at that point, the 1 or 2 hours of sleep and relaxation were gone. There was no way I could relax and sleep. I was angry. I was anxious. And I was so tired.

When exhaustion hits, take a look at the postpartum plan you filled out while pregnant. Which friends or family members can you ask to come over to hold and feed the baby so you can take a nap? Call or text that person.

Many times, hiring a postpartum doula or night nurse can be super helpful. This allows you (and your partner) to get a full night's sleep as the doula or nurse will feed, change, and care for the baby during that 8-hour period. Of course, this decision is based on your financial means and comfort level with having someone stay in your home.

## Infant Sleep Safety

Please be wary of the information in baby sleep training books and online trainings, as well as the information from the internet. Infant sleep depends entirely on the age, weight, and developmental age of your baby. As pediatricians, we do not recommend any sleep training earlier than 4 to 6 months of age. If you have specific questions, please discuss them with your pediatrician before sleep training your baby.

Remember:

- The safest place for your baby is in his or her own sleep space, such as a crib, bassinette, or pack-n-play.
- Remember the ABCs: alone-back-crib
  - A: Babies should sleep ALONE
  - B: Babies should sleep on their BACK
  - C: Babies should sleep in a CRIB, their own space that is uncluttered
- Approximately 3,500 babies die of sudden infant death syndrome yearly in the United States, most commonly between 1 and 4 months of age. This includes accidental suffocation/asphyxia, and undetermined deaths.

## POSTPARTUM MOOD AND ANXIETY DISORDERS

Another issue you need to be aware of is postpartum anxiety and depression. Mothers frequently ask me why they can't rest when the baby sleeps. Or a mom will say that she keeps watching her infant while she sleeps to make sure she is OK. One mom told me that she would put her hand on the baby's chest to make sure she was still breathing.

If you are unable to rest or sleep while the baby sleeps, this may be a red flag. If you are one of my mamas who is struggling with excessive worry about the baby or are anxious about something happening to your sleeping baby, you may be dealing with postpartum anxiety. As I said in Chapter 9, you are *not* alone, as postpartum depression/anxiety is one of the most common complications of childbirth. If you are experiencing any of these feelings, you need to tell someone you trust, whether that is your spouse, mother, aunt, or friend. And then you need to make an appointment with your obstetrician. If you have a history of anxiety or depression and have mental health services in place, please call your psychologist/therapist immediately. Just because you've had a baby does not mean you can neglect your mental health. Remember, your body and brain are connected, so you need to take care of both.

For my mothers who are struggling with a mood disorder that is getting worse with the sleep deprivation of having a newborn, please call the obstetrician or health care professional who delivered your baby. Also, please discuss this issue with your baby's pediatrician. Even though mom is not our patient, as pediatricians we care about you too, as your health and well-being directly impact the baby's health and well-being. If you are feeling overwhelmed or have questions, please ask for help. You are not alone.

If breastfeeding your newborn is exacerbating your anxiety or depression by worsening your sleep, then I am here to give you permission to stop breastfeeding. Moms tell me that when they decided to stop nursing, they felt much better. I have heard this from moms after their first baby as well as after their third. For many moms who struggle with underlying mental health issues, exclusively nursing is not always the best option. And that is OK. As discussed in Chapter 9, your mental health, and this includes sleep, is of the utmost importance.

## IMPORTANT NOTE FOR
## MY READERS

I want you to know, mama, that you are doing a great job. Remember to give yourself grace and forgiveness. And while so much of this time is a blur as you are feeling tired, let me tell you this. You have a lifetime ahead of you with your baby, as he or she smiles, crawls, and begins to walk. As your baby says a first word and tries food for the first time. There will be bumps along the way, but remember that your baby feels and knows how much you love them. However, you need to take care of yourself. Remember to ask for help and surround yourself with those who will be a positive part of your journey.

Being a pediatrician and providing evidence-based information was of utmost importance to me in writing this book. My primary intention was to talk to you—a mother or a mother-to-be—as another mom who has experienced much of what you are feeling. That was key for this book. Not to give isolated advice and evidence in a bubble, but rather to convey information through real-life situations that many, if not all, mothers have experienced at one time or another. Thank you.

Writing this book has allowed me to turn my passion into a reality, and I thank each and every one of you for reading this. I truly hope that this book has helped and will continue to help you on this journey of motherhood. During the initial phases of writing, my incredibly patient editor commented that throughout the book, I identify myself as a mother first and physician second, and she asked me why. Honestly, I had no idea that I was writing that way; my words just came naturally. But to answer, I will tell you this. While being a pediatrician and giving evidence-based information was of utmost importance to me in writing this book, first and foremost, my intention was to talk to you as someone who has experienced much of what you are feeling. To me, that was key for this book.

# Index